Virtual Medical Office

for

Bonewit-West, Hunt, Applegate:
Today's Medical Assistant:
Clinical and Administrative Procedures
Second Edition

Study Guide prepared by

Tracie Fuqua, BS, CMA (AAMA)
Program Director
Medical Assistant Program
Wallace State Community College
Hanceville, Alabama

Textbook by

Kathy Bonewit-West, BS, MEd
Coordinator and Instructor
Medical Assistant Technology
Hocking College
Nelsonville, Ohio
Former Member, Curriculum Review Board of the
American Association of Medical Assistants

Sue A. Hunt, MA, RN, CMA (AAMA)
Professor Emeritus
Medical Assisting Program
Middlesex Community College
Lowell, Massachusetts

Edith Applegate, MS
Professor of Biological Sciences
Kettering College
Kettering, Ohio

Software developed by

Wolfsong Informatics, LLC
Tucson, Arizona

D1621553

ELSEVIER
SAUNDERS

ELSEVIER
SAUNDERS

3251 Riverport Lane
Maryland Heights, Missouri 63043

VIRTUAL MEDICAL OFFICE FOR
BONEWIT-WEST, HUNT, APPLEGATE:
TODAY'S MEDICAL ASSISTANT: CLINICAL AND ADMINISTRATIVE PROCEDURES
SECOND EDITION

ISBN: 978-1-4557-4864-8

Copyright © 2013, 2009 by Saunders, an imprint of Elsevier Inc.

Notice

ISBN: 978-1-4557-4864-8

Executive Content Strategist: John Dolan
Senior Content Development Specialist: Jennifer Bertucci
Publishing Services Manager: Pat Joiner-Myers
Senior Project Manager: Stephen Bancroft

Printed in the United States of America

Last digit is the print number: 9   8   7   6   5   4   3

Table of Contents

Getting Started

■ LOGIN AND ENROLLMENT INSTRUCTIONS

Please check with your instructor prior to registering to verify whether you are required to enroll in the instructor's *Virtual Medical Office* course on Evolve. If so, your instructor will provide you with your course ID and you will use the steps under **Instructor-Led Course** on the following page.

SELF-STUDY COURSE

1. To access your *Virtual Medical Office*, go to http://evolve.elsevier.com/Bonewit/Today/.
2. Select the **Simulations—VMO** tab and click **Register for These Simulations** to begin the one-time-only registration process.
3. Select **I already have an Access code** and enter the code located on the inside front cover of this Study Guide exactly as it appears.
4. Click **Register**.
5. If you already have an Evolve account or have previously requested products from Evolve, provide your case-sensitive username and password in the Returning User area and click **Login**. If you do not have an Evolve account, provide your desired password for the account in the New User area and click **Continue**. Provide the required profile information and click **Continue**.
6. Read the Registered User Agreement. Check **Yes, I accept this agreement** and then click **Submit**.
7. A screen confirming your enrollment will appear. Click **My Home**.
8. This product will be added to your Evolve account in the My Content area located on the left-hand side of the Evolve homepage. Click to expand the **Simulations—VMO** heading and then click the link titled **Bonewit-West: Today's Medical Assistant, 2nd Edition**.
9. Click **Simulations—VMO** to access your activities.
10. Your case-sensitive account information will be e-mailed to you. Please note your account information. If needed, you can request your account information at any time by clicking on **I forgot my login information** on the Evolve homepage.
11. Bookmark this page (http://evolve.elsevier.com/student) to easily log in and access your *Virtual Medical Office* in the future.

Instructor-Led Course

1. Go to http://evolve.elsevier.com/enroll.
2. Enter the **Course ID** provided to you by your instructor and click the arrow button.
3. Verify that the course information is correct and check **Yes, this is my course**.
4. Select **I already have an Access code** and enter the code located on the inside front cover of this Study Guide exactly as it appears.
5. Click **Register**.
6. If you already have an Evolve account or have previously requested products from Evolve, provide your case-sensitive username and password in the Returning User area and click **Login**. If you do not have an Evolve account, provide your desired password for the account in the New User area and click **Continue**. Provide the required profile information and click **Continue**.
7. Read the Registered User Agreement. Check **Yes, I accept this agreement** and click **Submit**.
8. A screen confirming your enrollment will appear. Click **Get Started** or **My Home**.
9. This product will be added to your Evolve account in the My Content area located on the left-hand side of the Evolve homepage. Click to expand the **Simulations—VMO** heading and then click **Bonewit-West: Today's Medical Assistant, 2nd Edition**.
10. Click **Course Documents** and then click **Simulations—VMO** to access your activities.
11. Your case-sensitive account information will be emailed to you. Please note your account information. If needed, you can request your account information at any time by clicking on **I forgot my login information** on the Evolve homepage.
12. Please bookmark this page (http://evolve.elsevier.com/student) to easily log in and access your *Virtual Medical Office* in the future.

■ SUPPORT INFORMATION

Visit the Evolve Support portal at http://evolvesupport.elsevier.com to access the Evolve Knowledge Base, Downloads, and Support Ticket System. Live Evolve Support is also available 24/7 by calling 1-800-222-9570.

GETTING SET UP

■ **TECHNICAL REQUIREMENTS**

To use an Evolve online product, you will need access to a computer that is connected to the Internet and equipped with web browser software that supports frames. For optimal performance, it is recommended that you have speakers and use a high-speed Internet connection. Dial-up modems are not recommended for *Virtual Medical Office*.

WINDOWS®

Windows PC
Windows XP, Windows Vista™
Pentium® processor (or equivalent) @ 1 GHz (Recommend 2 GHz or better)
800 x 600 screen size
Thousands of colors
Soundblaster 16 soundcard compatibility
Stereo speakers or headphones
Internet Explorer (IE) version 6.0 or higher
Mozilla Firefox version 2.0 or higher

MACINTOSH®

Mozilla Firefox version 2.0 or higher

■ **WEB BROWSERS**

Supported web browsers include Microsoft Internet Explorer (IE) version 6.0 or higher and Mozilla Firefox version 2.0 or higher.

Whichever browser you use, the browser preferences must be set to enable cookies and the cache must be set to reload every time.

■ SCREEN SETTINGS

For best results, your computer monitor resolution should be set at a minimum of 800 x 600. The number of colors displayed should be set to "thousands or higher" (High Color or 16 bit) or "millions of colors" (True Color or 24 bit).

WINDOWS

1. From the **Start** menu, select **Settings**, then **Control Panel**.
2. Double-click on the **Display** icon.
3. Click on the **Settings** tab.
4. Under **Screen resolution** use the slider bar to select **800 x 600 pixels**.
5. Access the **Colors** drop-down menu by clicking on the down arrow.
6. Select **High Color (16 bit)** or **True Color (24 bit)**.
7. Click on **Apply**, then **OK**.
8. You may be asked to verify the setting changes. Click **Yes**.
9. You may be asked to restart your computer to accept the changes. Click **Yes**.

MACINTOSH

1. Select the **Monitors** control panel.
2. Select **800 x 600** (or greater) from the **Resolution** area.
3. Select **Thousands** or **Millions** from the **Color Depth** area.

Enable Cookies

Browser	Steps
Internet Explorer (IE) 6.0 or higher	1. Select **Tools → Internet Options**. 2. Select **Privacy** tab. 3. Use the slider (slide down) to **Accept All Cookies**. 4. Click **OK**. -OR- 3. Click the **Advanced** button. 4. Click the check box next to **Override Automatic Cookie Handling**. 5. Click the **Accept** radio buttons under **First-party Cookies** and **Third-party Cookies**. 6. Click **OK**.
Mozilla Firefox 2.0 or higher	1. Select **Tools → Options**. 2. Select the **Privacy** icon. 3. Click to expand Cookies. 4. Select **Allow sites to set cookies**. 5. Click **OK**.

Set Cache to Always Reload a Page

Browser	Steps
Internet Explorer (IE) 6.0 or higher	1. Select **Tools → Internet Options**. 2. Select **General** tab. 3. Go to the **Temporary Internet Files** and click the **Settings** button. 4. Select the radio button for **Every visit to the page** and click **OK** when complete.
Mozilla Firefox 2.0 or higher	1. Select **Tools → Options**. 2. Select the **Privacy** icon. 3. Click to expand Cache. 4. Set the value to "0" in the **Use up to: __ MB of disk space for the cache** field. 5. Click **OK**.

Plug-Ins

 Adobe Acrobat Reader—With the free Acrobat Reader software, you can view and print Adobe PDF files. Many Evolve products offer student and instructor manuals, checklists, and more in this format!

Download at: http://www.adobe.com

 Apple QuickTime—Install this to hear word pronunciations, heart and lung sounds, and many other helpful audio clips within Evolve Online Courses!

Download at: http://www.apple.com

 Adobe Flash Player—This player will enhance your viewing of many Evolve web pages, as well as educational short-form to long-form animation within the Evolve Learning System!

Download at: http://www.adobe.com

 Adobe Shockwave Player—Shockwave is best for viewing the many interactive learning activities within Evolve Online Courses!

Download at: http://www.adobe.com

 Microsoft Word Viewer—With this viewer Microsoft Word users can share documents with those who don't have Word, and users without Word can open and view Word documents. Many Evolve products have testbank, student and instructor manuals, and other documents available for downloading and viewing on your own computer!

Download at: http://www.microsoft.com

Virtual Medical Office Quick Tour

Welcome to *Virtual Medical Office* (VMO), a virtual office setting in which you can work with multiple patient simulations and also learn to access and evaluate the information resources that are essential for providing high-quality medical assistance.

VMO's medical office is called Mountain View Clinic. Once you have signed in to Mountain View Clinic, you can access the Reception area, Exam Room, Laboratory, Office Manager area, and Check-Out area, as well as a separate room for Billing and Coding.

■ BEFORE YOU START

Make sure you have your textbook nearby when you use VMO. You will want to consult topic areas in your textbook frequently while working online and using this Study Guide.

■ HOW TO SIGN IN

- Access the simulation on the Evolve resource page for your textbook. See the **Getting Started** instructions on page 1 of the Study Guide for information on accessing your Evolve resources.
- Enter your name on the medical assistant identification badge. The name entered here will print out on your performance summary reports.
- Click **Start Simulation**.

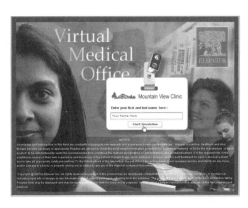

- This takes you to the office map screen. Across the top of this screen are photos of patients available for you to follow throughout their office visit.

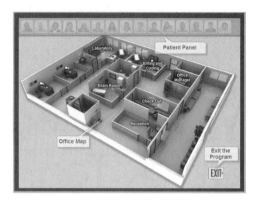

■ PATIENT LIST

1. **Janet Jones (age 50)**—Ms. Jones has sustained an on-the-job injury. She is in pain and impatient. By working with Ms. Jones, students will learn about managing difficult patients, as well as the requirements involved in workers' compensation cases.

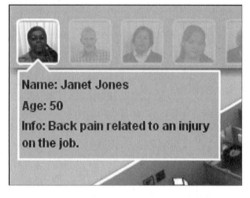

2. **Wilson Metcalf (age 65)**—A Medicare patient, Mr. Metcalf is being seen for multiple symptoms of abdominal pain, nausea, vomiting, and fever. He is seriously ill and might need more specialized care in a hospital setting.

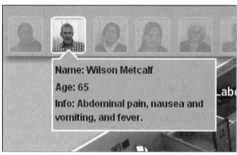

3. **Rhea Davison (age 53)**—An established patient with chronic and multiple symptoms, Ms. Davison does not have medical insurance.

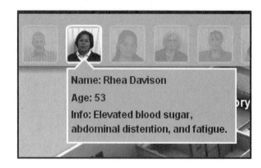

4. **Shaunti Begay (age 15)** — A new patient, Shaunti Begay is a minor who has an appointment for a sports physical. Upon arrival, Shaunti and her family learn that Mountain View Clinic does not participate in their health insurance.

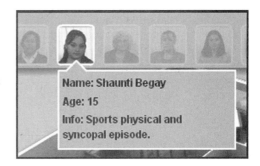

Name: Shaunti Begay

Age: 15

Info: Sports physical and syncopal episode.

5. **Jean Deere (age 83)** — Accompanied by her son, Ms. Deere is an established Medicare patient being evaluated for memory loss and hearing loss.

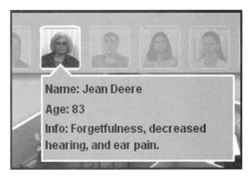

Name: Jean Deere

Age: 83

Info: Forgetfulness, decreased hearing, and ear pain.

6. **Renee Anderson (age 43)** — Ms. Anderson scheduled her appointment for a routine gynecologic exam but exhibits symptoms that suggest she is a victim of domestic violence.

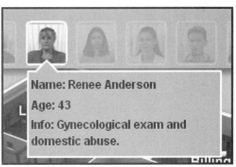

Name: Renee Anderson

Age: 43

Info: Gynecological exam and domestic abuse.

7. **Teresa Hernandez (age 16)** — Teresa is a minor patient who is unaccompanied by a parent for her appointment. She is seeking contraceptive counseling and STD testing.

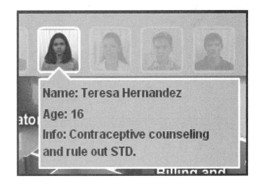

Name: Teresa Hernandez

Age: 16

Info: Contraceptive counseling and rule out STD.

8. **Louise Parlet (age 24)** — Ms. Parlet is an established patient being seen for a pregnancy test and examination. She will also need to be referred to an OB/GYN specialist.

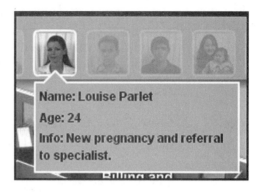

9. **Tristan Tsosie (age 8)** — A minor patient accompanied by his older sister and younger brother, Tristan is having a splint and sutures removed from his injured right arm.

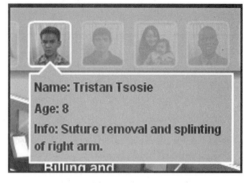

10. **Jose Imero (age 16)** — Jose is a minor patient who is scheduled for an emergency appointment to have the laceration on his foot sutured.

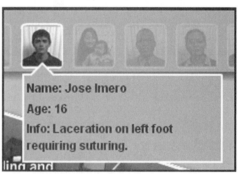

11. **Jade Wong (age 7 months)** — Jade and her parents are new patients to Mountain View Clinic. Jade needs a checkup and updates to her immunizations. Her mother does not speak English.

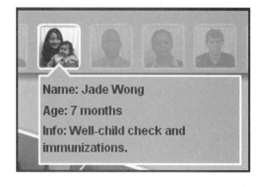

12. **John R. Simmons (age 43)** — Dr. Simmons is a new patient with a history of high blood pressure and recent episodes of blood in his urine.

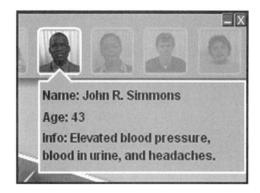

13. **Hu Huang (age 67)** — Mr. Huang developed a severe cough and fever after returning from a recent trip to Asia.

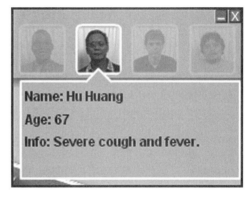

14. **Kevin McKinzie (age 18)** — Mr. McKinzie has made an appointment because of his nausea and vomiting. He is insured through the restaurant where he works.

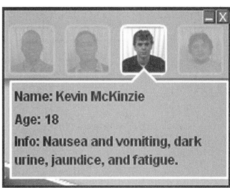

15. **Jesus Santo (age 32)** — Mr. Santo has been brought to the office as a walk-in appointment by his employer for leg pain and a fever. He has no insurance or identification, but his employer has offered to pay for the visit.

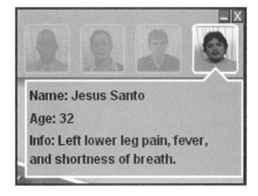

■ BASIC NAVIGATION

HOW TO SELECT A PATIENT

The list of patients is located across the top of the office map screen. Pointing your cursor at the various patients will highlight their photo and reveal their name, age, and medical problem (see examples in the illustrations on the previous pages). When you click on the patient you wish to review, a larger photo and description will appear in the lower left corner of the screen.

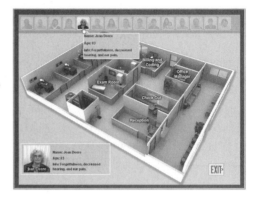

HOW TO SELECT A ROOM

After selecting a patient, use your cursor to highlight the room you want to enter. The active room will be shaded blue on the map. Click to enter the room.

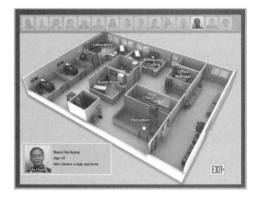

Note: You **must** select a patient before you are allowed access to any room.

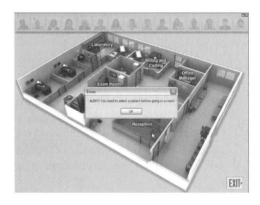

HOW TO LEAVE A ROOM

When you are finished working in a room, you can leave by clicking the exit arrow found at the bottom right corner of the screen.

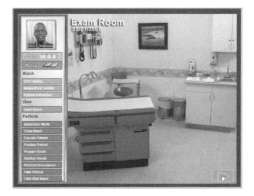

Leaving a room will automatically take you to the Summary Menu.

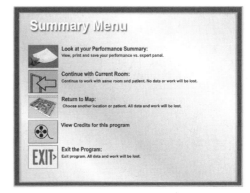

From the Summary Menu, you can choose to:

- **Look at Your Performance Summary**

  In each room there are interactive wizards or tasks that can be completed. The Performance Summary lets you compare your answers with those of the experts.

- **Continue with Current Room**

  This takes you back to the last room in which you worked. This option is not available if you have already reviewed your Performance Summary.

- **Return to Map**

  This reopens the office map for you to select another room and/or another patient.

- **View Credits for This Program**

  This provides a complete listing of software developers, publisher, and authors.

- **Exit the Program**

  This closes the *Virtual Medical Office* software. You will need to sign in again before you can use the program.

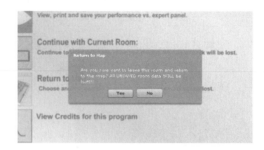

Note: If you choose to return to the office map, VMO alerts you that all unsaved room data will be lost. This means that any tasks completed in that room will be reset. Choose **Yes** to continue to the office map or **No** to return to the Summary Menu, where you can choose to continue working in the room or look at your Performance Summary.

HOW TO USE THE PERFORMANCE SUMMARY

If you completed any of the interactive wizards in a room, you can compare your answers with those of the experts by accessing your Performance Summary. This feature can be accessed after working in the Reception area, Exam Room, Laboratory, and Check Out area. The Performance Summary is not a grading tool, although it is valuable for self-assessment and review.

From the Summary Menu, click on **Look at Your Performance Summary**.

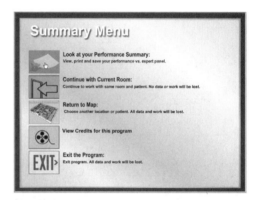

The complete list of tasks associated with the active room will appear with two columns showing the results of your choices. Your answers will appear in the column labeled **Your Performance**, and the answers chosen by the expert will appear in the **Expert's Performance** column. A check mark in both columns for a given task indicates that your answer matched the expert's answer. The Performance Summary can be saved to your computer or disk by clicking on the disk icon at the upper right side of the screen. The saved file can be printed or e-mailed to your instructor. A hard copy can also be printed without saving by clicking on the printer icon at the upper right corner of the screen.

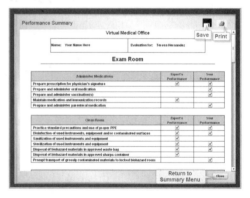

ROOM DESCRIPTIONS

All rooms can be entered at any time and in any order. You can follow a patient's visit from Reception to Check Out, or you can choose to observe patients at any point in their care. Below is a description of the information and activities that can be found in various rooms.

ALL ROOMS

- You can access the patient's medical record (Charts) and the office Policy Manual in all rooms.
- Each room has a sidebar Room Menu, from which you can choose to view documents, perform tasks, and watch videos.

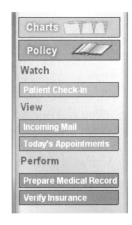

- The Reception area, Exam Room, and Check Out areas all feature videos in which you can watch the medical assistant interact with other Mountain View Clinic personnel and patients. Within the video screen you have a variety of options for navigating. Hover your cursor over the controls and status bar along the bottom of the video screen to reveal how each functions. By clicking various controls, you can play the video, pause it, forward or rewind using the scroll bar, and adjust the volume. Pressing the square stop button will stop the video and return the scroll bar to the beginning. Close the video screen by clicking on the **X** in the upper right corner of the screen.

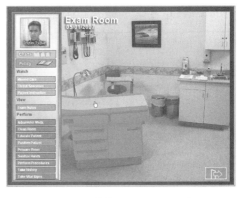

- Almost all rooms have **View** and **Perform** options on the Room Menu (*Note:* The Billing and Coding area does not have any Perform functions). These tasks can be completed either by clicking on the task description in the Room Menu or by clicking on the corresponding object in the room area. (For example, during an exercise, if you are required to perform the task of sanitizing your hands, the instructions may be worded as "Click on **Sanitize Hands** under Perform on the Room Menu," or you may simply be asked to "Click on the **Sink**." Both routes take you to the same task.) As you move your cursor over each item connected to one of the tasks on the View or Perform menu, both the object and the corresponding task in the Room Menu will highlight and become active. (*Note:* All corresponding pairs of instruction cues are listed in the individual room descriptions on the following pages.)

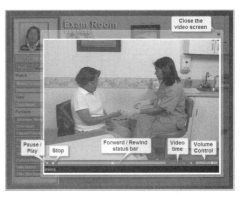

RECEPTION

In the Reception area, you can choose:

- **Charts**—Look at the patient's chart. *Note:* For new patients, there will be no information available in the chart at this time, although you do have the option of assembling a new medical record.
- **Policy**—Open the office Policy Manual and review the established administrative, clinical, and laboratory policies for Mountain View Clinic. Within the Policy Manual you will also find the Coding and Billing Manual.
- **Watch**—Watch a video of the patient's arrival. Each patient is shown checking in at the front desk so that you can observe the procedures typically performed by the receptionist and consider some of the various problems that might arise.
- **View**—Look at the Incoming Mail for the day by clicking on the stack of letters located on the **Stackable Trays** on the Reception desk. Review Today's Appointments by clicking on the **Computer** on the Reception desk to open up the day's schedule.
- **Perform**—Perform tasks at the Reception desk that are part of an administrative medical assistant's duties. Practice how to Prepare a Medical Record for a patient by clicking on the **Medical Record** file folder on the Reception desk. Verify Insurance for a patient by clicking on the **Insurance Card** on the counter at the Reception desk window.

EXAM ROOM

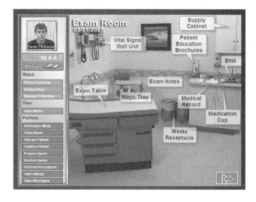

- **Charts** and **Policy**—Access the patient's chart and the office Policy Manual.
- **Watch**—View videos of different parts of the patient's exam. Observe the actions of the medical assistants in the videos and critique the competencies demonstrated.
- **View**—Review the physician's documented findings for the current visit in the Exam Notes. These notes are added to the full Progress Notes in the patient's chart as the patient continues on to Check Out. This can be accessed by clicking on the **Exam Notes** on the Exam Room counter.
- **Perform**—Perform multiple tasks that are required of a clinical medical assistant, such as preparing the room for the exam, taking vital signs and patient history, and properly positioning the patient for an exam. For each task listed under Perform on the Room Menu (cues on the left below), a corresponding object in the room area (cues on the right below) can also be clicked to access and perform the task:
  - **Administer Meds = Medication Cup**
  - **Clean Room = Waste Receptacles**
  - **Educate Patient = Patient Education Brochures**
  - **Position Patient = Exam Table**
  - **Prepare Room = Supply Cabinet**
  - **Sanitize Hands = Sink**
  - **Perform Procedures = Mayo Tray**
  - **Take History = Medical Record**
  - **Take Vital Signs = Vital Signs Wall Unit**

LABORATORY

- **Charts** and **Policy**—Access the patient's chart and the office Policy Manual.
- **View**—View the laboratory's log of specimens sent out for testing. Opportunities to practice filling out laboratory logs are included in the Study Guide exercises. This can be accessed by clicking on the **Lab Log Binder** on the Laboratory counter.
- **Perform**—Perform specific tasks as needed in the laboratory, such as collecting and testing specimens. These interactive wizards walk you through the steps for collecting and testing specimens ordered by the physician as part of the patient's exam. Access the Collect Specimens function by clicking on the **Specimen Collection Tray** on the counter. Complete the Test Specimens task by clicking on the **Specimen Analyzer**, also on the laboratory counter.

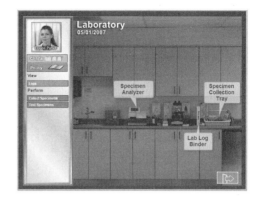

CHECK OUT

- **Charts** and **Policy**—Access the patient's chart and the office Policy Manual.
- **Watch**—Watch a video of the patient checking out of the office at the end of the visit. Observe the administrative medical assistants as they schedule follow-up appointments, accept payments, and manage the various duties and problems that may arise.
- **View**—The Encounter Form for each patient's visit can be accessed by clicking on the **Encounter Form** on the clipboard on the Check Out desk.
- **Perform**—Certain patients will require a return visit to the office. Schedule their follow-up appointments as needed by clicking on the **Computer** on the Check Out desk.

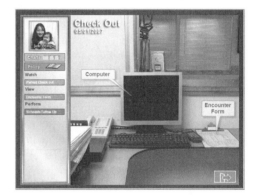

BILLING AND CODING

- **Charts** and **Policy**—Access the patient's chart and the office Policy Manual.
- **View**—Review the outstanding balances on various patient accounts and assess when to implement different collection techniques by clicking on the **Aging Report** on the left side of the Billing and Coding desk. Use the patient's **Encounter Form** on the right side of the desk to determine whether the proper procedures were followed to ensure accurate billing and coding. The office's **Fee Schedule** (on the wall to the left of the computer) is used to calculate the proper charges for the patient's visit.

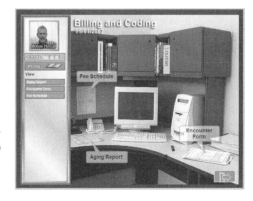

OFFICE MANAGER

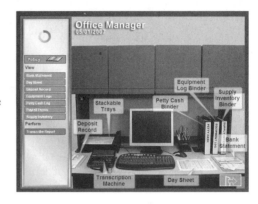

- **Policy**—View the office Policy Manual. Note that patient charts are not available from the Office Manager area.
- **View**—A variety of financial and administrative documents are available for viewing in the Office Manager area to practice managing office finances. Corresponding clues are listed below (menu terms on left; object cues on right):
  - **Bank Statement = Bank Statement** green file folder
  - **Day Sheet = Day Sheet** to the right of the computer keyboard
  - **Deposit Record = Deposit Record** to the left of the **Transcription Machine**
  - **Equipment Logs = Equipment Log Binder**
  - **Petty Cash Log = Petty Cash Binder**
  - **Payroll Forms =** located in the **Stackable Trays**
  - **Supply Inventory = Supply Inventory Binder**
- **Perform**—A recorded medical report is included for transcription practice with full player controls. This can be accessed by clicking on the Transcription Machine to the left of the computer keyboard.

■ EMBEDDED ERRORS

The individual lessons and patient scenarios associated with the *Virtual Medical Office* program were designed to stimulate critical thinking and analytical skills and to help develop the competencies you will be tested on as part of your course work. Thus deliberate errors have been embedded into each of the 15 patient scenarios and in the Billing and Coding and Office Manager activities. Many of the exercises in the Study Guide draw attention to these errors so that you can learn to recognize when and why a correction needs to be made, as well as how to correct it. Other errors have not been specifically addressed, and you may discover them as you work through the various rooms and tasks. These errors, when found, provide great learning opportunities to further develop the essential critical thinking and decision-making skills needed for professional work in the clinical office.

The following icons are used throughout the Study Guide to help you quickly identify particular activities and assignments:

 Reading Assignment—tells you which textbook chapter(s) you should read before starting each lesson

 Writing Activity—certain activities focus on written responses such as filling out forms or completing documentation

 Online Activity—marks the beginning of an activity that uses the *Virtual Medical Office* simulation software

 Online Instructions—indicates the steps to follow as you navigate through the software

 Reference—indicates questions and activities that require you to consult your textbook

 Time—indicates the approximate amount of time needed to complete the exercise

See the Evolve site for a Detailed Office Tour.

The Health Care System and the Professional Medical Assistant

Reading Assignment: Chapter 1—The Health Care System
Chapter 2—The Professional Medical Assistant

Patient: Rhea Davison   (*Note:* The first exercise does not involve Rhea Davison, but you have to choose a patient to access the clinic rooms.)

Learning Objectives:

- Identify the flow of activity in ambulatory care.
- Identify the various types of health care professionals and responsibilities of medical staff members in the outpatient medical office.
- Understand the difference in CMA (AAMA) and RMA credentials and the accrediting body that awards these credentials.
- Recognize professional and unprofessional behaviors.
- Understand the importance of following the office policy in regard to HIPAA standards.

Overview:

In this lesson you will learn about the flow of patient care and the essential guidelines for providing a professional and welcoming office environment for patients. You will observe the checking in of a patient and review the importance of patient confidentiality.

Exercise 1

Online Activity—Flow of Patient Care and Office Environment

 10 minutes

- Sign in to Mountain View Clinic and review the office map.

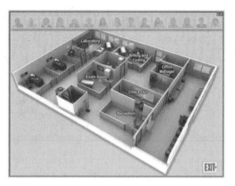

1. The patient list, which appears above the office map, shows the various patients who will be seen at Mountain View Clinic. Because there are multiple patients coming to the clinic to

    receive treatment, Mountain View Clinic is best described as an _____ care office.

2. Listed below are some of the rooms used by Mountain View Clinic. Based on what you have read in the textbook chapter, identify the order in which these rooms will be used for patient care.

Room	Order of Use
_____ Exam Room	a. First
_____ Laboratory	b. Second
_____ Reception	c. Third
_____ Check Out	d. Fourth

3. Which of the following items are necessary to have in a waiting room and reception area? Select all that apply.

_____ Weight scale with height bar

_____ Telephone

_____ Hazardous waste container

_____ Appointment book or computer for scheduling

_____ Patient charts

_____ Thermometer

_____ Mail

_____ Chairs

_____ Patient information and HIPAA forms

_____ Blood pressure cuff

_____ Reading material

Exercise 2

Writing Activity—Medical Specialties

10 minutes

1. The physicians at Mountain View Clinic may refer patients to specialists or for outpatient services that are not provided at the clinic. Match the following specialists with the service they provide.

Specialist	**Role in Health Care**
_____ Pediatrician	a. Provides anesthesia during surgery and other procedures
_____ Plastic surgery specialist	b. Specializes in the care of the ear, nose, throat, head, and neck
_____ Dermatologist	
_____ Immunologist	c. Specializes in conditions of the skin
_____ Physiatrist	d. Provides genetic counseling, prenatal diagnosis, and diagnostic procedures and treatment for individuals with genetically linked diseases
_____ Medical genetics specialist	
_____ Otolaryngologist	e. Specializes in the treatment and rehabilitation of patients with disabling conditions, such as spinal cord injury and stroke.
_____ Anesthesiologist	
	f. Specializes in the care of children from birth to adolescence.
	g. Provides surgical and nonsurgical treatment of physical defects of various areas of the body.
	h. Treats adults and children with allergies and problems of the immune system.

Exercise 3

Online Activity—Staff Member Responsibilities and Professionalism

 20 minutes

- From the patient list at the top of the office map, select **Rhea Davison**.

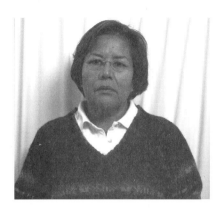

- On the office map, click on **Reception**.

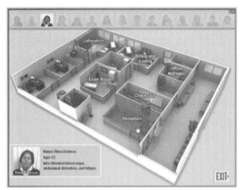

- To open the Policy Manual, click on **Policy** from the menu on the left side of the screen.

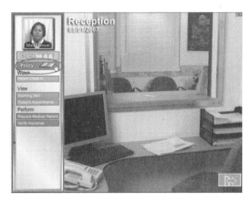

- When the Policy Manual opens, click on **Policy Manual** on the left and then type "job descriptions" in the search bar.
- Click on the magnifying glass and read through the job descriptions identified for Mountain View Clinic.
- After reading the job descriptions, type "HIPAA" in the search bar and click on the magnifying glass. Read the office policy on the Health Insurance Portability and Accountability Act (HIPAA) of 1996.

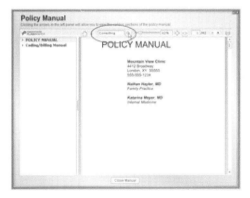

1. Match the specific duties listed below to the appropriate job title of the person who performs those duties. (*Hint:* You may use job titles more than once.)

Duties	**Job Title**
_____ Prepares patients and rooms to be used for exams, treatments, minor surgeries, and diagnostic tests	a. Office Manager
_____ Assembles all patient records for each day's appointments	b. Clinical Medical Assistant
_____ Schedules employees' work assignments	c. Administrative Medical Assistant
_____ Monitors compliance with all federal, state, and local statutes	d. Biller/Coder
_____ Performs CLIA-waived diagnostic tests	
_____ Files all insurance claims according to appropriate third-party guidelines	
_____ Transcribes dictated medical documents	
_____ Mails monthly accounts receivable statements	
_____ Obtains managed care precertifications for patient procedures and/or treatments	
_____ Handles incoming and outgoing mail	
_____ Sanitizes and sterilizes instruments	
_____ Prepares travel itineraries for physicians	
_____ Schedules mandatory inservices and staff meetings	

→ • Click on **Close Manual** to return to the Reception desk.

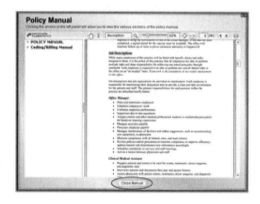

- Remain in the Reception area with Rhea Davison and select **Patient Check-In** to watch the video of Ms. Davison's arrival at Mountain View Clinic.

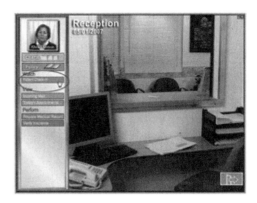

- At the end of the video, click on the **X** in the upper right corner of the screen to return to Reception.

In the video, the medical assistant discusses the CMA (AAMA) credential. However, the RMA is another credential that is recognized on a national level. (*Note:* The CMA credential must now be written as CMA (AAMA) to be distinguished from other CMA credentials that are not certified medical assisting credentials.)

2. Look up the CMA (AAMA) and RMA credentials and name the organizations that award these credentials.

3. Earlier, when you watched the video of Rhea Davison's check-in, what information did Kristin, the receptionist, neglect to collect from Ms. Davison?

4. What was your feeling about Kristin's behavior and the issue of confidentiality just before the arrival of the office manager?

5. In the video, the office manager appeared to be upset with Ms. Davison; however, do you think she was (or should have been) more upset with Kristin than with Ms. Davison? Explain your answer.

6. The office manager explained the need to follow HIPAA policy and the need for confidentiality of medical records. What did you think about the office manager's attitude and demeanor as she discussed the matter of confidentiality?

7. Why does the office manager need to explain the HIPAA policy in such a specific manner?

Critical Thinking Question

8. If you were at your clinical rotation and an office staff member violated HIPAA policy, how would you respond, as a student in this environment?

LESSON 2

Ethics and Law for the Medical Office

Reading Assignment: Chapter 3—Ethics and Law for the Medical Office

Patient: Wilson Metcalf

Learning Objectives:

- Recognize a potential liability problem and identify possible solutions.
- Identify breaches of medical ethics and etiquette at Mountain View Clinic.
- Determine the appropriate actions or behaviors to ensure that medical ethics and etiquette standards are met.

Overview:

In this lesson you will become familiar with the Policy Manual at Mountain View Clinic. You will recognize any unprofessional behaviors of the medical assistant and identify any medical ethical and etiquette errors made in providing care to the patient. The ethical and legal aspects of confidentiality are addressed.

Exercise 1

Online Activity—General Liability

20 minutes

- Sign in to Mountain View Clinic.
- Select **Wilson Metcalf** from the patient list.

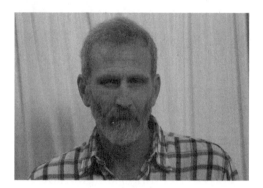

- On the office map, click on **Reception**.

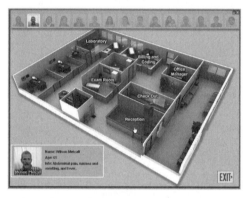

- Click on **Policy** to open the office Policy Manual.

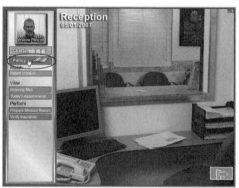

- Expand the Policy Manual's table of contents by clicking on the arrow next to Policy Manual on the menu on the left side of the screen.

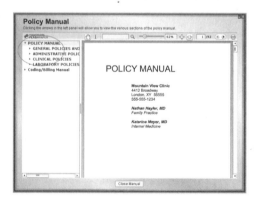

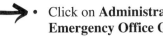

- Click on **Administrative Policies** and then on **Emergency Office Guidelines**. Read pages 17-19 of the Policy Manual.
- Click on **Close Manual** to return to the Reception desk.

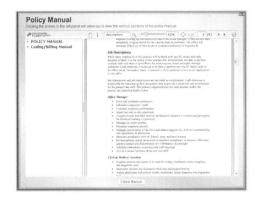

- Click on **Patient Check-In** (under Watch) to view the video of Mr. Metcalf's arrival at Mountain View Clinic.

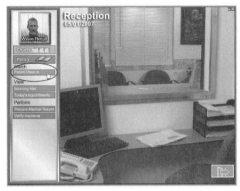

1. As you watched the video, what did you observe about Mr. Metcalf's condition?

2. Based on your observations, was it appropriate for Kristin to keep Mr. Metcalf waiting at the counter while she completed the check-in process? Explain your answer.

3. What was the rationale for Kristin to close the window? Was it appropriate for her to close the window at this time? Why or why not?

4. Did Kristin leave herself and the practice open to any potential liability issue(s) in this scene? If so, describe the issue(s) you identified.

5. Describe any other potential liability issues involving any of the other medical staff appearing in this video.

6. If Mr. Metcalf had been injured as a result of his fall and the subsequent treatment by the office staff and he then chose to pursue legal action against the practice, who would be at risk for liability?
   a. The physicians, the practice, and all three medical assistants
   b. The practice, Charlie, and Kristin
   c. Only Charlie and Kristin
   d. Only Kristin

7. What alternative actions could Kristin and the office staff have taken to avoid the potential liability issue(s) already identified? List at least five actions.

➡ • Click the **X** on the video screen to close the video and return to the Reception desk.

Exercise 2

Online Activity—Breaches of Medical Ethics and Medical Etiquette

 10 minutes

- Remain in the Reception area with Wilson Metcalf as your patient. (*Note:* If you have exited the program, sign back in to Mountain View Clinic and select Wilson Metcalf from the patient list.)
- Click on **Policy** to open the office Policy Manual.
- Click on **Policy Manual** (on the menu on the left), type "ethics" in the search bar, and then click on the magnifying glass.

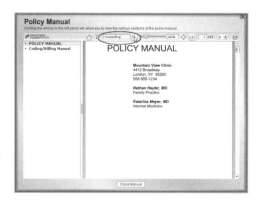

- Read the Work Ethics and Professional Behavior section in the Policy Manual.
- As you answer the following questions, you can leave the Policy Manual open. (*Note:* If necessary, click **Close Manual** to return to Reception and watch the Patient Check-In video again.)

1. The Professional Behavior section in the Policy Manual notes that employees are to show compassion and caring toward patients. Based on these guidelines, describe Kristin's interaction with Mr. Metcalf in the Patient Check-In video.

2. Below, list at least three medical ethics issues and three medical etiquette issues that you can identify from the Patient Check-In video with Mr. Metcalf.

Medical Ethics	Medical Etiquette

3. In addition to Kristin's comments about Mr. Metcalf needing soap, what did you notice about her nonverbal communications throughout the video?

4. Which patient right was violated in this scenario?
   a. The right to refuse treatment
   b. The right to be treated with respect and dignity
   c. The right to receive information about treatment suggested
   d. The right to select one's own physician

Exercise 3

 Writing Activity—Meeting Standards of Medical Ethics and Etiquette

10 minutes

In the previous exercise, you identified breaches of medical ethics and medical etiquette. In this exercise, you will determine the appropriate behaviors and actions that would have avoided these breaches and would have satisfied the office policy for professional behavior.

1. When Mr. Metcalf first appeared at Kristin's window to check in, which actions do you think would have demonstrated better medical ethics and etiquette? Select all that apply.

   _____ Ask Mr. Metcalf to supply all his new insurance information immediately.

   _____ Offer Mr. Metcalf a seat before asking for insurance information.

   _____ Ask Mr. Metcalf whether he is in pain and whether he requires assistance.

   _____ Notify a clinical medical assistant immediately that there is a patient in distress in the waiting room.

   _____ Notify the physician about Mr. Metcalf's distress.

   _____ Call 911.

   _____ Insist that Mr. Metcalf complete his new information form.

   _____ Close the window to protect the spread of possible infection while making copies of the insurance card.

   _____ Obtain all insurance information after Mr. Metcalf is placed in an examination room.

   _____ Move all patients out of the waiting room as soon as Mr. Metcalf arrives in the waiting room.

2. Which actions do you think would have demonstrated better medical ethics and etiquette from the time Mr. Metcalf fell to the floor until the end of the video? Select all that apply.

_____   Call 911.

_____   Notify the physician.

_____   Attempt to help Mr. Metcalf to a chair.

_____   Use the intercom to call for the red folder and additional assistance.

_____   Move the other patient in the waiting room away from Mr. Metcalf.

_____   Quietly document Mr. Metcalf's vital signs.

_____   Tell Mr. Metcalf that you think he will be okay.

_____   Reassure Mr. Metcalf that he will be cared for and that help is on the way.

3. What policy was violated when Kristin yelled for the red folder? (*Note:* Refer to the Policy Manual for help if you need it.)

Interacting with Patients

Reading Assignment: Chapter 4—Interacting with Patients

Patients: Janet Jones, Jade Wong

Learning Objectives:

- Differentiate between nonverbal and verbal communication.
- Identify factors that can interfere with effective communication.
- Correlate the existence of unmet needs to types of patient behavior in the health care setting.
- Explain the role of empathy in the relationship between the medical assistant and patients.
- Identify importance of sensitivity to cultural differences.
- Identify levels of human needs according to Maslow's Hierarchy of Needs.
- Understand different emotions patients experience when facing terminal illness.

Overview:

In this lesson you will learn about various communication methods medical assistants can use when faced with barriers such as anger, pain, and a difference in language. Human needs and emotions of patients who have terminal illness are also addressed.

Exercise 1

Online Activity—Verbal and Nonverbal Communication

 30 minutes

- Sign in to Mountain View Clinic.
- From the patient list, select **Janet Jones**.

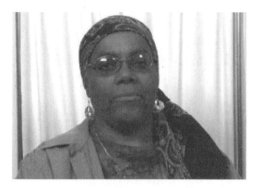

- On the office map, click on **Reception**.

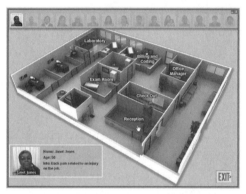

- Under the Watch heading, select **Patient Check-In** to view Janet Jones' arrival. Pause the video at the first fade-out.

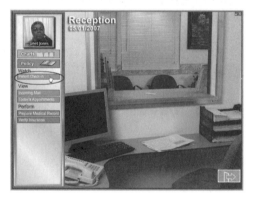

1. What verbal cues does Janet Jones give to Kristin about her mood and condition?

2. What nonverbal cues does Ms. Jones give to Kristin about her mood and condition?

3. What are Kristin's verbal and nonverbal responses to Ms. Jones?

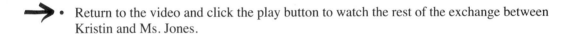

• Return to the video and click the play button to watch the rest of the exchange between Kristin and Ms. Jones.

4. In the second half of the video, has there been any change in Ms. Jones' attitude? If yes, describe what you observed and offer a rationale for her attitude change.

5. Has there been any change in Kristin's attitude or response towards Ms. Jones? If yes, describe what you observed and offer a rationale for the change.

6. Below, list at least three things Kristin did well in her communications with Ms. Jones. Then list three or more examples where she could improve in her future communications with patients.

Examples of Good Communication	Examples of Poor Communication/ Areas for Improvement

- Click **Close** to return to the Reception desk.
- Click the exit arrow and select **Return to Map**.

Exercise 2

Online Activity—Cultural Differences and Barriers to Communication

 15 minutes

- From the patient list, select **Jade Wong** as your patient. (*Note:* If you have exited the program, sign back in to Mountain View Clinic and select Jade Wong from the patient list.)

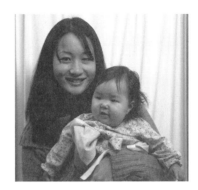

- Click to enter the **Exam Room**.

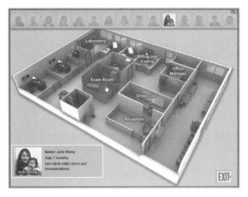

- Select **Charts** to open Jade's medical record. Review the Patient Information Form.

  1. What is the notation made on the line for Emergency Contact?

 • Click **Close Chart** to return to the Exam Room. Select **Well-Baby Visit** to watch the video.

  2. Who is the primary communicator for Jade Wong? Why do you think this is the case?

  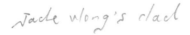 Jade wong's dad

3. Who does the medical assistant speak to as she explains the procedure? Is she communicating appropriately with Mr. and Mrs. Wong? Why or why not?

MR Wong auz Mrs Wong can Speak English

MR Wong is Mrs Wong's husband communication is effective auz they understand their language

4. The medical assistant in this video needed to overcome a barrier to communication. Listed below are some other potential barriers to communication. For each barrier, offer at least one possible way a medical assistant could overcome the barrier and ensure good communication with the patient.

Barriers to Communication	Recommended Solutions
Patient is deaf or hard of hearing.	
Patient is visually impaired or blind.	
Patient is in a wheelchair.	
Patient has a speech impediment.	

5. When a patient who speaks a foreign language needs to have minor office surgery,

_____ is required before the surgery can take place.

Exercise 3

Writing Activity—Basic Needs and Emotions Associated with Terminal Illness

15 minutes

1. Maslow's Hierarchy of Needs presents human needs as a pyramid, with each subsequent level of needs building on those already met. Match the columns below by placing the human needs in order from Level 1 (the most basic needs, which form the base of the pyramid) to Level 5 (the most complex needs, which form the top of the pyramid).

Human Needs		**Level**
C	Esteem and recognition	a. Level 1
D	Self-actualization	b. Level 2
E	Safety and security	c. Level 3
A	Love and belonging	d. Level 4
B	Physiologic needs	e. Level 5

2. Listed in the left column below are five emotional stages or responses to death or dying, as defined by Elisabeth Kübler-Ross. Match each emotional stage with its corresponding description of a patient diagnosed with a terminal illness.

Emotional Stage		**Patient Description**
C	Anger	a. Patient may try to give up something to gain something else.
A	Bargaining	b. Patient becomes silent and prefers to be alone.
D	Denial	c. Patient is frustrated and wonders "Why me?"
E	Acceptance	d. Patient is in a state of shock or disbelief.
B	Depression	e. Patient finds peace.

Medical Asepsis and the OSHA Standard

Reading Assignment: Chapter 17—Medical Asepsis and the OSHA Standard
- Microorganisms and Medical Asepsis
- OSHA Bloodborne Pathogens Standard

Patients: All Mountain View Clinic Patients

Learning Objectives:

- Discuss the rationale for handwashing versus hand sanitization.
- Identify the specific circumstances in which handwashing is appropriate.
- Identify the specific circumstances in which hand sanitization is appropriate.
- Examine the Policy Manual for policies regarding infection control for this office.
- Use the Internet to research information regarding hand hygiene.

Overview:

Handwashing has been a foundation of infection control for over a century. This practice is still essential today. Handwashing protects patients and health care workers from cross contamination. However, in certain cases designated by the Centers for Disease Control and Prevention (CDC), an alcohol-based hand rub may be used for hand sanitization. In this lesson we review the specific circumstances in which each of these means of hand hygiene is appropriate. After reviewing various online patient simulations, you will use the Mountain View Clinic Policy Manual and your own critical thinking skills to decide whether the medical assistant should wash his or her hands or use an alcohol-based hand rub in each case.

Exercise 1

Online Activity—Handwashing and Hand Sanitization

 35 minutes

- Sign in to Mountain View Clinic.
- From the patient list, select **Jean Deere**.
- On the office map, click on **Reception**.
- Next, click on **Policy** to open the Policy Manual.
- Select **Policy Manual** (from the menu on the left), type "handwashing" in the search bar, and click on the magnifying glass.
- Read the section of the Policy Manual regarding handwashing.

Since the Mountain View Clinic office follows the CDC guidelines, go to http://www.cdc.gov and search for "hand hygiene in health care settings." The CDC provides guidelines in PDF format. View these guidelines to learn the current recommendations. If you need assistance, your instructor can help you narrow your search based on current information or additional links.

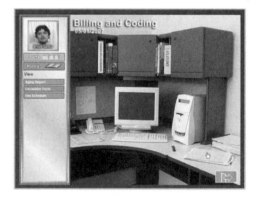

- Click **Close Manual** to return to the Reception area.
- On the Summary Menu, click **Return to Map** and select **Yes** on the pop-up window to return to the office map.
- From the patient list, select **Jesus Santo**. Mr. Santo was in the examination room just before Ms. Deere.
- On the office map, click on **Billing and Coding**.
- Click on the **Encounter Form** clipboard to find the diagnosis for Mr. Santo's visit.

1. Based on the diagnosis listed on the Encounter Form for Mr. Santo and your review of the CDC guidelines for hand hygiene, what would be the correct method of hand hygiene to use between patients?

• Click **Finish** to close the Encounter Form and return to the Billing and Coding area.
- Click the exit arrow in the lower right corner of the screen to exit the Billing and Coding area.
- On the Summary Menu, click **Return to Map** and select **Yes** on the pop-up window to return to the office map.
- From the patient list, select **Jean Deere**.
- On the office map, click on **Exam Room**.
- Under the Watch heading, click on **Room Preparation** and watch the video.

2. Why did the medical assisting extern need to perform handwashing before preparing the room for a patient?

3. According to CDC policy, if the patient seen before Jean Deere had not had a diagnosis with the possibility of disease transmission, what would have been the appropriate form of hand sanitization?

4. If the medical assistant wears gloves, is it necessary to perform hand hygiene when the gloves are removed before working with the next patient?

5. What potential risk do artificial fingernails or natural nails longer than ¼ inch present in the health care setting? (*Note:* For assistance, you may visit the CDC website at http://www.cdc.gov/mmwr/preview/mmwrhtml/rr5116a1.htm to view current CDC recommendations. Scroll down the page to find "Other Policies Related to Hand Hygiene: Fingernails and Artificial Nails.")

Critical Thinking Question

6. Laney will be starting her medical assisting externship in a few days. She has been advised that she will need to remove her artificial nails before she can begin working as an extern. Laney is upset about this requirement because the nails were expensive. She mentions to you that she doesn't understand why she needs to remove the nails since she'll be working with gloves on anyway. What would you say to Laney to convince her of the importance of having the artificial nails removed?

 • Click the **X** in the upper right corner to close the video and return to the Exam Room.

• Inside the Exam Room, click on the **Sink**. This will activate the Sanitize Hands task.

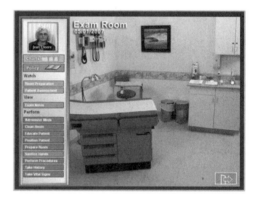

• Use the radio buttons to select the correct method of hand sanitization to be used after Jean Deere's examination.

• Click **Finish** to return to the Exam Room.

• Click the exit arrow in the lower right corner of the screen to exit the Exam Room.

• On the Summary Menu, click on **Look at Your Performance Summary**.

• Scroll down the Performance Summary to the Sanitize Hands section; compare your answers with those chosen by the experts.

• You may save and print the Performance Summary for your records or turn it in to your instructor. The icons for saving and printing the Performance Summary are located at the top right corner of the screen.

• Click **Close** to return to the Summary Menu.

• On the Summary Menu, click **Return to Map** and select **Yes** on the pop-up window to return to the office map.

• From the patient list, select **Louise Parlet**.

• On the office map, click on **Exam Room**.

• Under the Watch heading, click on **Infection Control** and watch the video.

Critical Thinking Question

7. Would it have been acceptable for the medical assisting extern to have cleaned the table without gloves if she had sanitized her hands before and immediately after disposing of the table paper and gown? Why or why not?

Critical Thinking Question

8. After the extern has cleaned the examination table and removed the gloves, what is the appropriate means of hand hygiene?

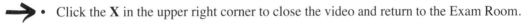

- Click the **X** in the upper right corner to close the video and return to the Exam Room.
- Click the exit arrow in the lower right corner of the screen to exit the Exam Room.
- On the Summary Menu, click **Return to Map** and select **Yes** on the pop-up window to return to the office map.

Exercise 2

Online Activity—Hand Sanitization with Possible Infectious Disease

20 minutes

- From the patient list, select **Kevin McKinzie**.
- On the office map, click on **Check Out**.
- Click on **Charts** to open Kevin McKinzie's medical record.
- Click on the **Patient Medical Information** tab and select **1-Progress Note** from the drop-down menu.

1. What is the possible diagnosis for this patient?

2. With this diagnosis, what would be the safest means of hand hygiene after patient care?

3. Indicate whether the following statement is true or false.

   _____ According to the CDC, the use of gloves is not necessary when good hand hygiene is used.

4. According to the CDC guidelines, when is handwashing always necessary in the medical office? (*Hint:* Refer to the textbook if you need help.)

5. According to the CDC guidelines, when may an alcohol-based hand rub be used for hand sanitization?

6. The CDC has recommended the use of alcohol-based hand rubs instead of handwashing in some instances. What are the advantages of alcohol-based hand rubs? (*Hint:* Refer back to the text if you need assistance.)

• Click **Close Chart** when finished to return to the Check Out area.
• Click the exit arrow in the lower right corner of the screen to exit the Check Out area.
• On the Summary Menu, click **Return to Map** and select **Yes** on the pop-up window to return to the office map.

Exercise 3

  Online Activity—Handwashing and Hand Sanitization

 45 minutes

For additional practice, you will review the Progress Notes of all the patients at Mountain View Clinic and decide whether hand sanitization with traditional handwashing or with an alcohol-based hand rub would be the better choice. Your instructor may assign all of the patients or just a few.

• From the patient list, select **Janet Jones**.
• On the office map, click on **Exam Room**.
• Inside the Exam Room area, click on the **Sink** to activate the Sanitize Hands task.
• Before completing this task, read the documentation regarding Janet Jones' visit by clicking on **Exam Notes** in the Room Menu.

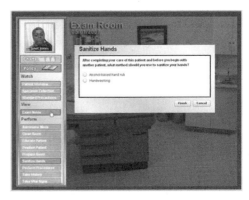

• Click **Finish** to close the Exam Notes and return to the Sanitize Hands window.
• Use the radio buttons to select the correct method of hand sanitization that should follow Ms. Jones' examination.
• Click **Finish** to return to the Exam Room.
• Click the exit arrow in the lower right corner of the screen to exit the Exam Room.
• On the Summary Menu, click on **Look at Your Performance Summary**.
• Scroll down the Performance Summary to the Sanitize Hands section and compare your answers with those chosen by the experts.

• You may save and print the Performance Summary for your records or turn it in to your instructor. The icons for saving and printing the Performance Summary are located at the top right corner of the screen.

• Click **Close** to return to the Summary Menu.

• On the Summary Menu, click **Return to Map** and select **Yes** on the pop-up window to return to the office map.

• Repeat these steps for all the patients at Mountain View Clinic and compare your answers with the experts.

• *Note:* If the expert chose alcohol-based hand rub and you chose handwashing, your choice might not be considered the preferred method, but it would still be acceptable because handwashing with running water and antibacterial soap would be effective as well.

Regulated Medical Waste

/OO **Reading Assignment:** Chapter 17—Medical Asepsis and the OSHA Standard
- OSHA Bloodborne Pathogens Standard
- Regulated Medical Waste

Patients: Shaunti Begay, Hu Huang, Tristan Tsosie

Learning Objectives:

- Recognize what materials are biohazardous.
- Describe the proper disposal of used medical equipment and supplies.
- Identify the proper practice of standard precautions.
- Understand how to apply Occupational Safety and Health Administration (OSHA) standards.
- Apply critical thinking skills to answer questions regarding biohazardous waste.
- Understand the importance of an infection control plan and its impact on preventing the spread of disease in the medical facility.

Overview:

This lesson discusses OSHA regulations concerning medical waste. You will learn to distinguish acceptable practices from those practices that could cause injury to patients and staff. Included in the practice of universal precautions are standard precautions, which include the appropriate disposal of biohazardous waste. (Note: Although medical asepsis, including handwashing, is an important factor in infection control, this topic is covered in another lesson and will not be addressed here.)

Exercise 1

 Online Activity—Infection Control in the Medical Office Using OSHA Standards

20 minutes

- Sign in to Mountain View Clinic.
- From the patient list, select **Shaunti Begay**.
- Click on **Policy** to open the office Policy Manual.
- Select **Policy Manual**, type "OSHA" in the search bar, and click on the magnifying glass.

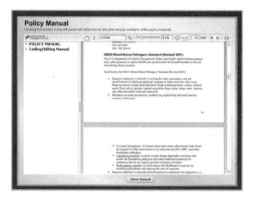

- Read the section of the Policy Manual regarding OSHA Bloodborne Pathogens.
- Keep the Policy Manual open to answer the following questions.

1. Name four body fluids that would be considered biohazardous waste in this medical office.

Critical Thinking Question

2. What additional body secretion is not included in the list of biohazardous waste?

3. What does the term *universal precaution* refer to?

4. What are work practice controls?

5. What are engineering controls?

6. What does *PPE* stand for?

7. Identify the procedures that, according to the standard, must be followed in regard to housekeeping. (*Hint:* Refer to your textbook if you need help.)

→ • Click **Close Manual** to return to the Exam Room.
  • Remain in the Exam Room with Shaunti Begay as your patient and continue to the next exercise.

Exercise 2

Online Activity—Application of OSHA Standards

30 minutes

- Under the Watch heading, click on **Immunizations** and watch the video.
- Pause the video at the first fade-out by clicking the pause button in the lower left corner of the video screen.

1. Did the medical assistant wear the proper PPE for giving an injection? Explain your answer.

2. Did the medical assistant properly handle the disposal of the gloves and waste from the injection?

3. Where did she dispose the used needle and syringe?

4. What engineering controls did you see in the video?

 • Click the **X** in the upper right corner to close the video and return to the Exam Room.
- Click the exit arrow in the lower right corner of the screen to exit the Exam Room.
- On the Summary Menu, click **Return to Map** and select **Yes** on the pop-up window to return to the office map.
- From the patient list, select **Hu Huang**.
- On the office map, click on **Reception**.
- Under the Watch heading, click on **Patient Check-In** to watch Hu Huang checking in to the clinic.

Critical Thinking Question

5. Mr. Huang has a productive cough when he approaches the reception area. He lays a contaminated tissue on the counter just before Kristin takes him to a room. Should she have left the area without disinfecting the counter? Explain your answer.

6. Explain the proper disposal of contaminated tissues.

7. Which of the following are proper steps in infection control that should be observed during the check-in of Mr. Huang? Select all that apply.

_____   Provide tissues as shown in the video.

_____   Allow Mr. Huang to stay in the waiting room.

_____   Throw the tissue in the trash at the desk so that the contamination cannot spread.

_____   Apply gloves before handling the used tissues.

_____   Provide Mr. Huang with a biohazard waste bag in which to dispose of any used tissues.

_____   Wash hands after disinfecting the counter.

_____   Don a gown and mask when caring for Mr. Huang.

Critical Thinking Question

8. Based on the video you watched, how do you think the patients in the waiting room felt when the medical assistant stated that Mr. Huang might have an infectious disease that could be spread to the other patients? Do you think Kristin handled the check-in procedure in an ethical manner? Explain your answer.

Critical Thinking Question

9. If Kristin had not placed the patient in the examination room, do you think patients would have complained verbally about Mr. Huang's persistent cough? Can you think of possible situations in which you could not move a patient into a separate room? Explain your answer.

10. Indicate whether each of the following statements is true or false.

a. _____ Because Mr. Huang laid his contaminated tissue on the counter, OSHA standards would require that Kristin disinfect the counter before allowing another patient to register.

b. _____ Ideally, after Mr. Huang laid his tissue on the counter, Kristin should have donned gloves and removed the tissue before moving the patient to a room.

c. _____ Ideally, in offices in which patients may have infectious diseases, a biohazard waste bag should be placed at the check-in window for situations similar to what you saw in the video.

d. _____ Ideally, the check-in desk should have nonsterile gloves available for removing biohazardous waste.

e. _____ Because Kristin did not touch the contaminated tissues, she does not need to sanitize her hands.

f. _____ The better method of sanitization of Kristin's hands would be handwashing with soap and water.

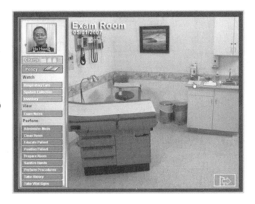

- Click the **X** in the upper right corner to close the video and return to the Reception area.
- Click the exit arrow in the lower right corner of the screen to exit the Reception area.
- On the Summary Menu, click **Return to Map** and select **Yes** on the pop-up window to return to the office map.
- On the office map, click on **Exam Room**.
- Click on the **Exam Notes** file folder to read the documentation regarding Hu Huang's visit.

- Click **Finish** to close the Exam Notes and return to the Exam Room.
- Click on the **Waste Receptacles** in the Exam Room.
- Use the checkboxes to select the appropriate steps necessary to clean the Exam Room after Hu Huang's examination.
- Click **Finish** to return to the Exam Room.
- Click the exit arrow in the lower right corner of the screen to exit the Exam Room.
- On the Summary Menu, click on **Look at Your Performance Summary**.
- Scroll down the Performance Summary to the Clean Room section and compare your answers with those chosen by the experts.
- You may save and print the Performance Summary for your records or turn it in to your instructor. The icons for saving and printing the Performance Summary are located at the top right corner of the screen.
- Click **Close** to return to the Summary Menu.
- On the Summary Menu, click **Return to Map** and select **Yes** on the pop-up window to return to the office map.

Exercise 3

Online Activity—Applying Knowledge of Federal Regulations (OSHA)

 15 minutes

- From the patient list, select **Tristan Tsosie**.
- On the office map, click on **Exam Room**.
- Under the Watch heading, click on **Throat Specimen** and watch the video, observing the infection control measures.

1. Which of the following PPE did Cathy use when she obtained a throat culture? Select all that apply.

   _____ Sterile gloves

   _____ Nonsterile gloves

   _____ Face shield

   _____ Sterile gown

   _____ Disposable gown

   _____ Goggles

2. Indicate whether each of the following statements is true or false.

   a. _____ Cathy followed OSHA policy regarding the PPE needed for obtaining a throat culture.

   b. _____ The supplies used to collect the throat specimen should be disposed in the biohazard waste container.

   c. _____ The gown and mask may be used again with another patient since Tristan did not cough.

   d. _____ The PPE used by Cathy must be provided by her employer.

   e. _____ If the biohazard bag is not full at the end of the day, it would be acceptable to wait and add tomorrow's waste and then discard the bag when it is full.

   f. _____ Each medical office must have its own infection control system.

   g. _____ Compliance with OSHA standards is required by law.

3. Do you think Cathy handled the use of PPE in an acceptable manner when talking with Tristan? Explain your reasoning.

 • Click the **X** in the upper right corner to close the video and return to the Exam Room.

• Click the exit arrow at the lower right corner of the screen to exit the Exam Room.

• On the Summary Menu, click **Return to Map** and then click **Yes** at the pop-up menu to return to the office map or click **Exit the Program**.

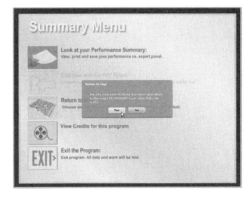

Sterilization and Disinfection

/OO **Reading Assignment:** Chapter 18—Sterilization and Disinfection
Chapter 25—Minor Office Surgery
- Surgical Asepsis
- Instruments Used in Minor Office Surgery

Patient: Jose Imero

Learning Objectives:

- Identify the reasons for checking instruments for repairs before wrapping.
- Identify the reasons for performing sanitization before sterilization.
- Discuss the need for double-wrapping some items before sterilization.
- Describe the use of indicator strips in sterilization techniques and quality control.
- Identify the items needed for wrapping articles for sterilization.
- Identify the steps required for wrapping items for sterilization.
- Understand the reasons for performing sanitization before sterilization.
- State the reason for using indicator strips in sterilization techniques and quality control.
- Sequence the steps required for wrapping items for sterilization.
- Match causes of improper sterilization with problems that will result if the proper technique is not followed.
- Discuss the storage requirements for items that have been autoclaved.
- Identify instruments frequently used in minor office surgery.

Overview:

In this lesson you will learn the difference between sanitization and sterilization. You will observe Danielle, the medical assisting extern, prepare instruments for sterilization and discuss the proper steps that must be followed to ensure effective sterilization.

Exercise 1

  Online Activity—Sanitation and Sterilization

45 minutes

1. What does it mean to *sanitize* equipment?

2. What does it mean to *sterilize* equipment?

3. List the seven general steps in the sanitization procedure of instruments.

4. Indicate whether the following statement is true or false.

_____ Before sanitization, instruments should be rinsed in cool water and dried thoroughly.

5. Which of the following should be used during the sanitization of instruments that have blood on them? Select all that apply.

_____ Hot water initially

_____ Low-sudsing detergent

_____ Warm water initially

_____ Hot water to rinse

_____ Cold water initially

_____ High sudsing detergent

_____ Brush

_____ Warm water to rinse

6. What should the medical assistant wear while sanitizing instruments?

Critical Thinking Question

7. If you are unable to sanitize an instrument immediately, what can you do to prevent the body fluid and debris from drying on the instrument?

 • Sign in to Mountain View Clinic.
  • From the patient list, select **Jose Imero**.
  • On the office map, click on **Exam Room**.
  • Under the Watch heading, click on **Sterilization Techniques** and watch the video.

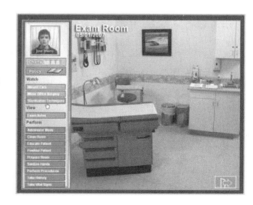

8. In the video, Charlie asks Danielle whether she has checked the instruments to ensure that the "instruments approximate." What does it mean for an instrument to *approximate*? (*Hint:* Use a dictionary or other source if needed to answer this question.)

9. In the video, Charlie asks Danielle whether she has compared the instruments to see whether everything that is needed is on the tray. Why do you think he asked this question?

10. Why do you think Charlie asks whether the indicator strip is "in date?"

11. What is the reason for the chemical indicator strip?

12. Which of the following supplies are needed when wrapping instruments and equipment for sterilization? Select all that apply.

    _____ Sterilization paper, muslin, or sterilization pouches

    _____ Permanent marker

    _____ Sterilization indicator strip

    _____ Pen

    _____ Autoclave tape

    _____ Pencil

13. After the autoclave cycle is complete, does the color of the autoclave tape indicate whether or not the package is sterile? Support your answer.

14. Charlie told Danielle to begin with the wrapping material in a diamond shape. Why is this important when wrapping articles for sterilization?

15. After Danielle completes the autoclave procedure, where should she store the sterilized articles?

16. Indicate whether each of the following statements is true or false.

a. _____ When instruments with movable parts are being wrapped, the joint should be closed to prevent moisture from adhering to the instrument and causing rust.

b. _____ When instruments with sharp edges are being wrapped, the edges should first be wrapped in gauze.

c. _____ All instrument packs should be autoclaved for the same amount of time, regardless of the size of the package or the contents.

d. _____ Autoclave tape indicates that the package is sterile.

e. _____ Any ballpoint pen is acceptable for labeling a package for the autoclave.

f. _____ The first fold made in wrapping an instrument should be the fold closest to your body at the bottom of the package.

17. Which of the following should appear on the label of a wrapped article for the autoclave? Select all that apply.

_____ Type of instrument or equipment found in package

_____ Indicator strip inside

_____ Date of sterilization

_____ Initials of person preparing package

_____ Expiration date for the package

18. Match the columns below to show the correct sequence of actions in wrapping an instrument for autoclaving.

Action		Order of Sequence
_____	Fold the top corner of the wrap toward the center and fold a tab.	a. Step 1
_____	Fold the bottom corner of the wrapping material toward the center and fold a tab.	b. Step 2
		c. Step 3
_____	Place autoclave tape across the outside corner.	
_____	Flip the instrument in the wrap until it is a neat package.	d. Step 4
		e. Step 5
_____	Fold each side of the wrap into the center, leaving a tab on each side.	

→ • Click the **X** in the upper right corner to close the video and return to the Exam Room.
  • Click the exit arrow in the lower right corner of the screen to exit the room.
  • On the Summary Menu, click **Return to Map** and select **Yes** at the pop-up menu to return to the office map or click **Exit the Program**.

Exercise 2

Writing Activity—Identifying Instruments Used in the Medical Office

15 minutes

1. Identify the following types of scissors by matching each image with its name.

Images   **Names**

_____ 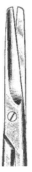   a. Lister bandage scissors

                                              b. Littauer suture scissors straight

                                              c. Mayo dissecting scissors curved

                                              d. Mayo dissecting scissors straight

                                              e. Operating scissors sharp-blunt

_____ 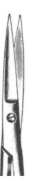   f. Operating scissors sharp-sharp

                                              g. Operating scissors straight

_____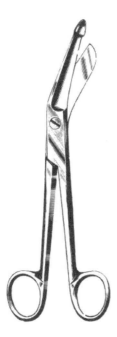

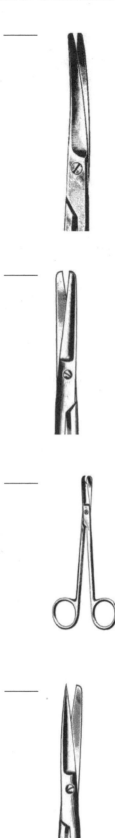

2. Identify the following types of thumb forceps by matching each image with its name.

Images   **Names**

_____ 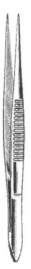   a. Adson dressing forceps

                                                       b. Plain splinter forceps

                                                       c. Standard tissue forceps

                                                       d. Straight thumb forceps

_____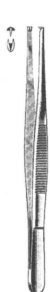

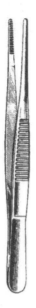

3. Identify the following types of ring-handled forceps by matching each image with its name.

Images

Names

_____

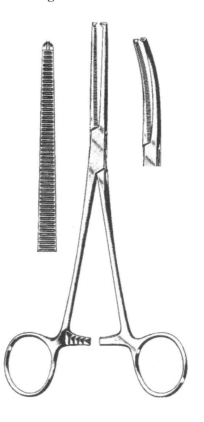

a. Allis tissue forceps

b. Foerster sponge forceps

c. Halsted mosquito hemostatic forceps

d. Kelly hemostatic forceps

e. Ochsner-Kocher hemostatic forceps

f. Rochester-Pean hemostatic forceps

_____

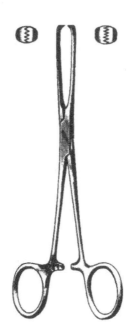

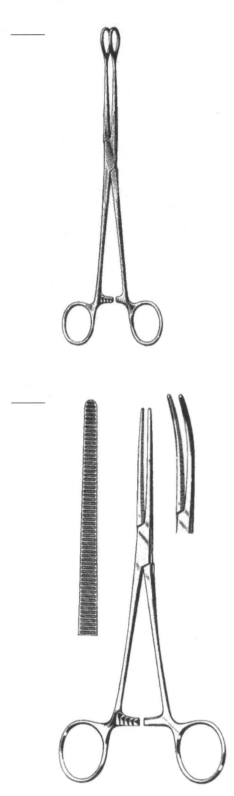

_____

_____

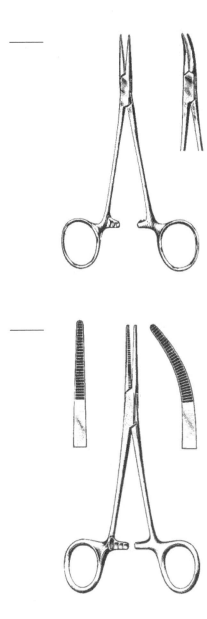

Obtaining Vital Signs

_____

/OO **Reading Assignment:** Chapter 19—Vital Signs

Patients: All Mountain View Clinic Patients

Learning Objectives:

- State the normal range for body temperature, based on the site used to measure the reading.
- Identify conditions or factors that alter body temperature.
- Identify the three terms used to describe the characteristics of the patient's pulse.
- Describe conditions or factors that alter pulse rate and rhythm.
- Identify terms related to respiration.
- State the normal respiratory rate ranges, depth, and rhythm.
- Describe conditions that alter respiratory function.
- State the normal ranges for blood pressure.
- Describe conditions or factors that alter blood pressure, including age-related factors.
- Discuss what is meant by hypertension, prehypertension, and normal blood pressure.

Overview:

This lesson is intended to provide an understanding of the importance of correctly obtaining vital signs. Dr. John R. Simmons is a college professor who has a history of hypertension. Teresa Hernandez is a teenage patient. You will be using the Policy Manual to decide what steps you need to include in patient care to be in compliance with the physician's standing orders for these patients. After reviewing the information and answering questions about normal ranges for vital signs, you will be asked to check the vital signs of the patients at Mountain View Clinic and recognize which patients do not have normal vital sign results.

Exercise 1

Online Activity—Obtaining Temperature, Pulse, and Respiration

 30 minutes

- Sign in to Mountain View Clinic.
- From the patient list, select **Teresa Hernandez**.
- On the office map, click on **Exam Room**.
- Click on **Policy** to open the office Policy Manual.
- Select **Policy Manual**, type "standing orders" in the search bar, and click on the magnifying glass.

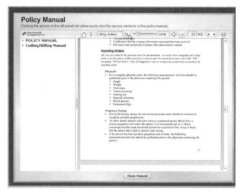

- Read the Standing Orders section of the Policy Manual.
- Click **Close Manual** to return to the Exam Room.

1. What are Mountain View Clinic's standing order instructions regarding vital signs and physical examinations?

2. List seven factors that can affect or cause variations in a patient's body temperature.

3. If you were to check the temperature of a 6-year-old child who had just been playing outside in the summer sun, would you expect his or her temperature to be slightly elevated? Why or why not?

Critical Thinking Question

4. What course of action could you take to double-check and ensure that the child's body temperature was higher as a result of activity rather than illness?

5. Which of the following temperature readings would be considered normal in an adult patient?
   a. Oral: 98.6° F
   b. Axillary: 97.6° F
   c. Aural: 98.6° F
   d. Options a, b, and c

6. Which of the following statements about temperature are true? Select all that apply. (*Hint:* Use your critical thinking skills.)

   _____ The medical assistant must be aware of the normal ranges of temperature for screening patient vital signs.

   _____ Temperature ranges are the same for all ages.

   _____ Equipment used for obtaining temperature readings should be checked on a regular basis to ensure proper working condition.

   _____ All temperature readings have the same baseline, regardless of the body site where they are taken.

   _____ It is acceptable to take a body temperature reading immediately after a patient has eaten, smoked, or exercised.

   _____ When taking vital signs, the medical assistant should have an organized order in which to obtain the readings.

   _____ Usually, vital signs are documented in this order: temperature, pulse, and then respirations.

   _____ Body temperature is a measure of the balance between the heat produced in the body and the heat lost from the body.

   _____ The normal body temperature range is from 97° to 99° F.

   _____ Fever is defined as any temperature above 98.6° F.

7. An average body temperature of 98.6° F is considered _____, whereas a

   temperature below 97° F is considered subnormal or _____. If the patient

   has a temperature above 100.4° F, he or she is considered to have a _____.

   If the temperature measures between 99° and 100.4° F, it is considered a

   _____.

8. A person with fever is described as _____, whereas a person without

   fever is called _____.

9. Match each of following normal temperatures with the age group to whom it applies.
   (*Note:* Some of the items in the right column include a temperature range or the site where
   taken. Be sure to note these factors.)

Age Group	**Normal Temperature**
_____ Newborn	a. 97.6° F
_____ Older adult	b. 96.8° F (oral site)
_____ 5-year-old child (oral site)	c. 97° to 100° F (axillary site)
_____ Adult (axillary site)	d. 98.6° F

10. What is specifically being measured when the pulse rate is obtained?

11. Which of the following factors may affect the pulse? Select all that apply.

    _____ Metabolism

    _____ Age

    _____ Physical activity

    _____ Emotional states

    _____ Gender

    _____ Fever

    _____ Weather conditions

    _____ Medications

    _____ Respiratory rate

12. Which of the following are acceptable sites for obtaining a pulse rate? Select all that apply.

_____ Across the abdomen

_____ Popliteal area

_____ Radial and ulnar surfaces

_____ Temporal area

_____ Axillary area

_____ Femoral area

_____ Apical area

_____ Brachial area

_____ Carotid areas

_____ Dorsalis pedis

_____ Anterior tibial area

13. Match each of the following average pulse rates with the group of individuals to whom the rate applies. (*Hint:* Refer to your textbook to check your work after making your choices.)

Average Pulse Rate (bpm)   **Group**

_____ 90-140   a. Newborns

_____ 40-60   b. Toddlers

_____ 120-160   c. Children (3 to 6 years)

_____ 67-80   d. School-age children (6 to 8 years)

_____ 60-100   e. Adolescents and adults

_____ 80-110   f. Adult (60 years and older)

_____ 75-105   g. Athletes

14. Pulse measurement is described by _____, _____, and

_____.

15. What is meant by *dysrhythmia*?

16. When discussing pulse volume, a _____ indicates a fast, weak pulse,

    whereas a _____ indicates an extremely strong, full pulse.

17. Why is the respiratory rate considered a vital sign?

18. Which of the following factors may affect respirations? Select all that apply.

    _____ Age

    _____ Physical activity

    _____ Eye color

    _____ Disease processes

    _____ Emotional state

    _____ Gender

    _____ Medications

    _____ Fever

19. Match each of the following respiratory sounds to its definition.

Sound		**Definition**
_____	Rhonchi	a. High-grating sound similar to that of leather pieces rubbing together, heard on auscultation
_____	Wheezes	
_____	Crackles	b. Dry or wet intermittent sound that varies in pitch; similar to the sound of hairs rubbing together
_____	Pleural friction rub	c. Deep, low-pitched rumbling sound; heard more on expiration
		d. High whistling musical sound; heard on both inspiration and expiration

20. Match each of the following average respiratory rate ranges with the age group to which it applies.

**Average Respiratory
Rate Range (breath/min)**   **Age Group**

_____ 12-20   a. Infants

_____ 23-35   b. Toddlers (1 to 3 years)

_____ 30-40   c. Preschool-age children (3 to 6 years)

_____ 18-26   d. School-age children

_____ 20-30   e. Adolescents and adults

21. The taking in of oxygen is called _____, whereas the

    breathing out of carbon dioxide is called _____.

    Together, these two mechanisms are considered one _____.

22. Match each of the following terms with its definition.

Definition   **Term**

_____ Dyspnea that is relieved by standing or   a. Apnea
        sitting positions
                                                     b. Sleep apnea
_____ Bluish discoloration of the skin
                                                     c. Adventitious sounds
_____ Difficult breathing or shortness of breath
                                                     d. Orthopnea
_____ Absence of respiration
                                                     e. Dyspnea
_____ Abnormal breath sounds
                                                     f. Cyanosis
_____ Absence of respirations during periods of rest

23. Indicate whether each of the following statements is true or false.

    a. _____ When an aural temperature is taken on a toddler, the auricle should be
                 pulled down and back.

    b. _____ When an aural temperature is taken on an adult, the auricle should be pulled
                 up and back to expose the tympanic membrane.

    c. _____ For all vital signs, the patient should be told what procedures are about to be
                 performed.

    d. _____ If you are taking a patient's pulse rate before counting the respiratory rate,
                 you should release the pressure from the patient's wrist before you count the
                 respirations.

    e. _____ Measuring a rectal temperature is a safe procedure for all patients.

f. _____ It is acceptable to obtain the pulse rate using the radial site on all patients.

g. _____ When pulse rate is being recorded, any deviation of rhythm or volume should be documented.

h. _____ When respiratory rate is being recorded, any deviation in rhythm or volume should be documented.

→ • Inside the Exam Room menu, click on the **Vital Signs Wall Unit**.

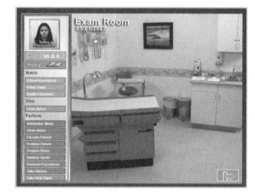

• Click **Take Blood Pressure**. Teresa Hernandez's blood pressure reading will appear in the box below.

• Repeat this step for all vital signs.

• Record each reading in the appropriate box at the bottom of the screen.

• If a result is abnormal, click to select the box that says, "Check if physician needs to be notified of abnormality."

24. Which, if any, of Teresa Hernandez's vital signs are *not* within normal limits?

25. Why would Teresa's systolic number not be considered prehypertensive? (*Hint:* Use Table 19-8 in the textbook if you need help.)

→ • Click **Finish** to return to the Exam Room.

• Click the exit arrow in the lower right corner of the screen to exit the Exam Room.

• On the Summary Menu, click on **Look at Your Performance Summary**.

• Scroll down the Performance Summary to the Take Vital Signs section and compare your answers with those chosen by the experts.

• You may save and print the Performance Summary for your records or turn it in to your instructor. The icons for saving and printing the Performance Summary are located at the top right corner of the screen.

• Click **Close** to return to the Summary Menu.
- On the Summary Menu, click **Return to Map** and select **Yes** at the pop-up menu to return to the office map.
- On the office map, click on **Check Out**.
- Click on **Charts** to open Teresa Hernandez's medical record.
- Click on the **Patient Medical Information** tab and select **1-Progress Notes** from the drop-down menu.

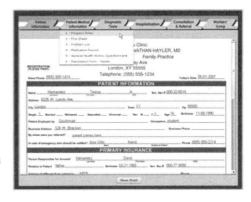

- Read the entire documentation of Teresa Hernandez's visit for this date.

26. Did the medical assistant obtain the necessary vital signs? Explain your answer.

Critical Thinking Question

27. Suppose Teresa arrives at the office and barely finishes signing in when you are ready to move her into the examination room. You immediately measure her pulse rate (148 bpm) and respiratory rate (36 breaths/min). While you are recording her chief complaint, Teresa mentions that she was out of breath when she arrived because the elevator in the building is out of order and she had to walk up 16 flights of stairs. Would these circumstances have any bearing on the readings you just obtained? What would be the appropriate procedure to follow in this instance?

 • When finished, click **Close Chart** to return to the Check Out area.
- Click the exit arrow in the lower right corner of the screen to exit the room.
- On the Summary Menu, click **Return to Map** and select **Yes** at the pop-up menu to return to the office map.

Exercise 2

Online Activity—Obtaining Blood Pressure Readings

20 minutes

1. What is specifically assessed by blood pressure measurements?

2. Why is the diastolic pressure always above zero?

3. Match each of the following terms with its definition.

Term	Definition
_____ Hypertension	a. Pressure on the walls of the arteries when the heart is at rest
_____ Pulse pressure	b. Blood pressure above 140/90
_____ Systolic pressure	c. Blood pressure below 90/60
_____ Hypotension	d. Pressure on the walls of the arteries when the heart is contracting
_____ Diastolic pressure	e. The difference between systolic and diastolic pressure

4. Which of the following factors affect blood pressure? Select all that apply.

_____ Time of day

_____ Age

_____ Environment

_____ Exercise

_____ Gender

_____ Emotions

_____ Body position

_____ Amount of sleep

_____ Medications

_____ Caffeine, recent meal, smoking

5. Define *normal blood pressure*, *prehypertensive state*, and *hypertension*.

6. What is the difference between stage 1 hypertension and stage 2 hypertension?

7. The equipment needed for obtaining blood pressure includes a _____

   and a _____.

8. Blood pressure cuffs come in the following sizes: _____,

   _____, and _____.

9. The sounds heard as blood pressure is being taken are called _____.

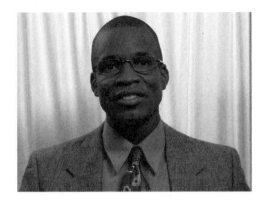

→ • From the patient list, select **John R. Simmons**. (*Note:* If you have exited the program, sign in again to Mountain View Clinic and select John R. Simmons from the patient list.)

- On the office map, click on **Check Out**.
- Click on **Charts** and select **1-Progress Notes** from the drop-down menu under the **Patient Medical Information** tab.
- Read the final documentation of Dr. Simmons' visit.

10. Are any of Dr. Simmons' vital sign results *not* within normal limits? If so, which?

11. According to American Heart Association standards, what is the interpretation of Dr. Simmons' documented blood pressure readings?

12. The blood pressure readings for Dr. Simmons were higher when taken the second time. What is a logical explanation for the difference?

13. Why do you think Dr. Meyer wants Dr. Simmons to take blood pressure readings at home and record them?

14. Notice that Dr. Simmons' blood pressure reading taken from the left arm is more elevated than the reading from the right arm. What is an explanation for this?

Exercise 3

Online Activity—Documentation of Vital Signs

40 minutes

1. Using today's date and time, accurately document the following scenario on the form below:

   Judy Marks (born 4/27/38) is taking medication for hypertensive disease and is seen at your clinic on a regular basis. Today, she has come in to have her vital signs checked by the medical assistant. Her pulse is 104 bpm, weak, and difficult to obtain, with a skipped beat every six beats. Her rate of breathing is 24 breaths/min and shallow. Her temperature is 97.6° F. Her blood pressure is 176/104 mm Hg in the left arm and 170/102 mm Hg in the right arm.

PATIENT'S NAME	Judy Marks		☒ FEMALE ☐ MALE		Date of Birth: 04/27/38
DATE	PATIENT VISITS AND FINDINGS				

ALLERGIC TO _____

ORDER #25-7133-01 • ©1999 BIBBERO SYSTEMS, INC. • PETALUMA, CA   TO REORDER CALL 800-BIBBERO (800-242-2376) OR FAX (800) 242-9330 MFG IN USA   PAGE ____ of ____

2. Which, if any, of the findings in question 1 need to be reported to the physician before Judy Marks leaves the clinic? Which findings are abnormal?

Now you will practice documenting information in the medical record of all of the patients at Mountain View Clinic. You will also make notations of any abnormal vital signs results. Review and follow the steps below for each patient, keeping track of any errors you make or any discrepancies between your work and that of the experts in your Performance Summary reviews.

- From the patient list, select **Janet Jones**.
- On the office map, click on **Exam Room**.
- Click on the **Vital Signs Wall Unit**.
- Click **Take Blood Pressure**. The patient's blood pressure reading will appear in the box just below this heading.

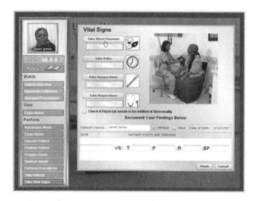

- Repeat this step for all vital signs.
- Record the readings in the appropriate boxes at the bottom of the screen.
- If any of the patient's results are abnormal, click to select the box that says, "Check if physician needs to be notified of abnormality." This will give you valuable practice in recognizing abnormal results that need to be brought to the physician's attention.
- Click **Finish** to return to the Exam Room.
- Click the exit arrow in the lower right corner of the screen to exit the room.
- On the Summary Menu, click on **Look at Your Performance Summary**.
- Scroll down the Performance Summary to the Take Vital Signs section and compare your answers with those chosen by the experts.
- You may save and print the Performance Summary for your records or turn it in to your instructor. The icons for saving and printing the Performance Summary are located at the top right corner of the screen.
- Click **Close** to return to the Summary Menu.
- On the Summary Menu, click **Return to Map** and select **Yes** at the pop-up menu to return to the office map.
- Now repeat the above steps for each of the remaining patients at Mountain View Clinic. Don't forget to compare your answer with the experts each time.

3. How did you do? Below, document any errors you made in transferring the information or any time you failed to notify the physician of abnormalities in normal readings.

Preparing and Maintaining Examination and Treatment Areas

/O⌒Ɔ **Reading Assignment:** Chapter 20—The Physical Examination
- Preparation of the Examining Room
- Preparation of the Patient

Patients: Jean Deere, Louise Parlet, Rhea Davidson, Jesus Santo

Learning Objectives:

- Describe the steps necessary in preparing an examination room for patient care.
- List supplies needed for a complete physical examination.
- Describe the steps necessary in cleaning the examination or treatment room after patient care
- Document patient vital signs and history in the patient medical record.

Overview:

This lesson identifies the supplies that are necessary in preparing an examination or treatment room for Jean Deere. After Ms. Deere has been examined by the physician, the examination or treatment room must be prepared for the next patient, Louise Parlet. A review of the necessary steps in infection control and disposal of biohazardous waste is presented, including questions addressing hand hygiene. You will also practice documenting in the patient medical record.

Exercise 1

**Online Activity—Preparing the Examination or Treatment Room for
Patient Care**

45 minutes

- Sign in to Mountain View Clinic.
- From the patient list, select **Jean Deere**.
- On the office map, click on **Exam Room**.
- Click on **Policy** to open the office Policy Manual.
- Type "room maintenance" in the search bar and click on the magnifying glass.
- Read the section of the Policy Manual regarding the preparation of examination and treatment rooms.
- Click **Close Manual** to return to the Exam Room.
- Under the Watch heading, click on **Room Preparation** and watch the video.
- Click the **X** in the upper right corner to close the video and return to the Exam Room.

1. The medical assisting extern washed her hands before setting up the examination or treatment room. Why is this an important step in room preparation?

2. The medical assistant extern asked Armeeta about Ms. Deere's symptoms. Why is this information important when preparing a room for the patient?

3. Indicate whether each of the following statements is true or false.

    a. _____ Infection control is important when preparing a room for a patient.

    b. _____ When preparing the room for a physical examination, all equipment must be in good working order, properly disinfected, and readily available for the physician's use during the examination.

    c. _____ The general cleanliness of the room has nothing to do with the patient's feelings about the overall medical office.

    d. _____ Waste receptacles in the examination or treatment room should be emptied frequently.

    e. _____ Biohazardous receptacles should be changed after providing any patient care that involves gross biohazard waste.

    f. _____ Sharps biohazard containers should be emptied daily.

g. _____ Equipment for the examination should be placed at easy access for the physician and, if possible, in the order of use.

h. _____ The medical assistant should know how to operate and care for the equipment found in the examination and treatment rooms.

i. _____ The room temperature should be determined by what is comfortable for the physician.

j. _____ All equipment in the examination room should be disposable.

k. _____ Proper disposal of equipment after use is an important factor in infection control.

l. _____ Improperly checked equipment and supplies may cause injury to a patient.

4. Match each of the following pieces of equipment with its description or purpose.

Equipment	Description or Purpose
_____ Sphygmomanometer	a. Light on a movable stand
_____ Drape and/or gown	b. Covering to reduce patient exposure and to provide modesty and warmth
_____ Basin	c. Used to test neurological reflexes
_____ Thermometer	
_____ Cotton-tipped applicator	d. Long stick with cotton cover used to collect specimens
_____ Tongue depressor	e. Used for wiping secretions
_____ Lubricant	f. Used to test hearing acuity
_____ Tape measure	g. Used to measure blood pressure
_____ Tuning fork	h. Used to measure temperature
_____ Percussion hammer	i. Used to auscultate sounds
_____ Speculum	j. Used to measure parts of the body
_____ Ophthalmoscope	k. Covering for hands for good infection control practices
_____ Otoscope	l. Container in which used instruments are placed
_____ Stethoscope	m. Flat wooden blade used to examine mouth and throat
_____ Tissues	n. Used to examine eyes
_____ Examination light	o. Used to open a body orifice
_____ Disposable gloves	p. Used to examine the ear canal
	q. Used to reduce friction

• Inside the Exam Room, click on the **Exam Notes** file folder to read the documentation regarding Jean Deere's visit.

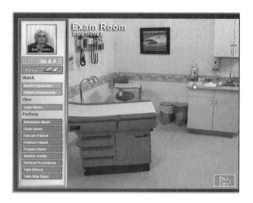

5. Armeeta was correct in assuming Dr. Meyer would want to perform an ear irrigation (lavage) and a pulse oximeter reading. What additional test did Dr. Meyer want done at this visit?

• Click **Finish** to close the Exam Notes and return to the Exam Room.
• Now click on the **Supply Cabinet** (this activates the Prepare Room task).
• Prepare the room by adding the supplies needed for Jean Deere's examination. From the Available Supplies list, click an item you think is needed. Then click **Add Item** to confirm your choice. The items you select will appear in the Selected Supplies box. When you click on an item, a photograph of the item will appear, which can be used for reference as you review your list of supplies. (Note: You can reopen the Exam Notes located in the lower left corner for reference as you make your selections.)
• If you wish to remove a chosen supply, highlight the supply in the Selected Supplies box and then click **Remove**.
• Repeat these steps until you are satisfied you have everything you need from the list.
• Once you are done making your selections, click **Finish** to return to the Exam Room.
• Next, activate the Take Vital Signs task by clicking on the **Vital Signs Wall Unit**.
• Click **Take Blood Pressure**. Jean Deere's blood pressure reading will appear in the box underneath.
• Repeat this for all vital signs.
• Record the readings in the appropriate boxes at the bottom of the screen.
• If any of Ms. Deere's results are abnormal, select the box that says, "Check if physician needs to be notified of abnormality."
• Once again, click **Finish** to return to the Exam Room.
• Click on the **Medical Record** clipboard (this activates the Take History task).

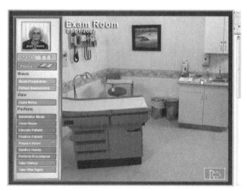

• Begin Ms. Deere's history by clicking on the **Ask** buttons to view her answers to questions regarding her medical history.

- Record the information in Ms. Deere's medical record in the box under "Document all findings below." Enter your name after your documentation, as requested by your instructor.

- At the bottom of the page, click **Next** to view additional questions and responses related to Ms. Deere's history.

- Click any boxes next to additional questions you think you would need to ask the patient.

- If requested by your instructor, print the information by clicking on **Print** at the bottom of the screen.

- Click **Finish** to close the Take History window and answer **Yes** at the pop-up window to return to the Exam Room.

- Click the exit arrow in the lower right corner of the screen to exit the room.

- On the Summary Menu, click on **Look at Your Performance Summary**.

- Scroll down the Performance Summary to find the sections that match the tasks you just performed: Prepare Room, Take Vital Signs, and Take History. For each task, compare your answers with those chosen by the experts.

- You may save and print the Performance Summary for your records or turn it in to your instructor. The icons for saving and printing the Performance Summary are located at the top right corner of the screen.

- Click **Close** to return to the Summary Menu.

- On the Summary Menu, click **Return to Map** and select **Yes** at the pop-up menu to return to the office map.

Critical Thinking Question

6. Based on your review of the Performance Summary, were there any items you selected that did not appear on the expert's list? Did you leave out any items on the expert's list? What impact could these discrepancies have on patient care?

Exercise 2

 **Online Activity—Maintaining the Examination or Treatment Room After
                    Patient Care**

 30 minutes

- From the patient list, select **Louise Parlet**.
- On the office map, click on **Exam Room**.
- Under the Watch heading, click on **Infection Control** and watch the video.
- Click the **X** in the upper right corner to close the video and return to the Exam Room.
- Click on **Policy** to open the office Policy Manual.
- Select **Policy Manual**, type "room maintenance" in the search bar, and click on the magnifying glass.
- Read the section of the Policy Manual regarding room maintenance.
- Keep the Policy Manual open to answer the following questions.

1. What does the Policy Manual indicate should be performed in the room after each patient has been seen?

2. During the video, did the medical assistant follow the Policy Manual procedures in regard to cleaning the room? Explain your answer.

3. During the video, did you see a break in infection control by the medical assisting extern? Explain.

4. Indicate whether each of the following statements is true or false.

a. _____ The medical assistant should use gloves, gown, and face shield when cleaning the examination room after a patient.

b. _____ The medical assistant should disinfect the table, supply tray, countertops, and table tops after each patient.

c. _____ Nondisposable supplies and equipment should be disinfected and properly stored when the room is cleaned.

d. _____ Nondisposable equipment should be sanitized and sterilized as necessary before storage.

e. _____ The office Policy Manual contains all information needed for the correct cleaning of a room after a patient's examination.

f. _____ The physician will inform the medical assistant of the items that must be discarded and those that should be sanitized and reused.

g. _____ Items such as ophthalmoscopes, otoscopes, and tuning forks do not require sanitization after use in patient care.

h. _____ Standard precautions should be followed when preparing and cleaning the examination or treatment room.

i. _____ If appointments are running behind schedule, the medical assistant knows that getting the appointment schedule back on time is more important than completely cleaning examination or treatment rooms after each patient is seen.

j. _____ It is permissible for the medical assistant to clean the examination or treatment room after the next patient has already been escorted into that room.

k. _____ Teamwork is essential in keeping the office neat, clean, and ready for patients.

Critical Thinking Question

5. What do you think would be the best action to take if you entered a room with a patient and discovered that the room had not been properly prepared?

- Click **Close Manual** to return to the Exam Room.
- To activate the Prepare Room task, click on the **Supply Cabinet**.
- Add the supplies needed for Louise Parlet's examination by clicking on each supply from the Available Supplies list and then clicking **Add Item** to confirm your choice. The items you select will appear in the Selected Supplies box. (*Note:* You can reopen the **Exam Notes** located in the lower left corner for reference as you make your selections.)

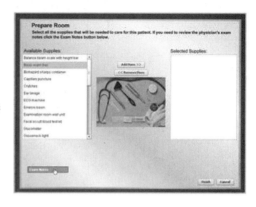

- If you wish to remove a chosen supply, highlight the supply in the Selected Supplies box and click **Remove**.
- Repeat these steps until you are satisfied you have everything you need from the list.
- Once you are done making your selections, click **Finish** to return to the Exam Room.
- Click on the **Vital Signs Wall Unit** to begin taking the patient's vital signs.
- Click **Take Blood Pressure**. Ms. Parlet's blood pressure reading will appear in the box underneath.
- Repeat this for all vital signs.
- Record the readings in the appropriate boxes at the bottom of the screen.
- If any of Ms. Parlet's results are abnormal, select the box that says, "Check if physician needs to be notified of abnormality."
- Click **Finish** to return to the Exam Room.
- Now click on the **Medical Record** clipboard to take Ms. Parlet's history.
- Click on the **Ask** buttons to view the patient's answers to questions regarding her medical history.

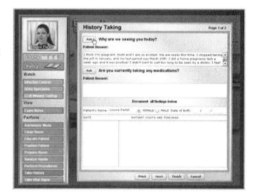

- Record the information in the patient's medical record in the box under "Document all findings below." Enter your name after your documentation, as requested by your instructor.
- At the bottom of the page, click **Next** to view additional questions and responses related to Ms. Parlet's history.
- Click any boxes next to additional questions you think you would need to ask the patient.
- If requested by your instructor, print the information by clicking on **Print** at the bottom of the screen.
- Click **Finish** to close the Take History window and answer **Yes** at the pop-up window to return to the Exam Room.
- Click the exit arrow in the lower right corner of the screen to exit the room.
- On the Summary Menu, click on **Look at Your Performance Summary**.
- Scroll down the Performance Summary to find the sections that match the tasks you just performed: Prepare Room, Take Vital Signs, and Take History. For each task, compare your answers with those chosen by the experts.
- You may save and print the Performance Summary for your records or turn it in to your instructor. The icons for saving and printing the Performance Summary are located at the top right corner of the screen.

→ • Click **Close** to return to the Summary Menu.

- On the Summary Menu, click **Return to Map** and select **Yes** at the pop-up menu to return to the office map.

Exercise 3

Online Activity—Cleaning the Treatment Room After Patient Care

 30 minutes

In this exercise you will have the opportunity to clean the examination room after different patients have been seen and treated. In each case, the proper steps to clean the room will depend on the individual patient's condition, needs, and treatment. First, you will clean the Exam Room after the physician has cared for Rhea Davison.

- From the patient list, select **Rhea Davison**.
- On the office map, click on **Exam Room**.
- Click on the **Exam Notes** file folder to read the documentation regarding Rhea Davison's visit.
- Click **Finish** to close the Exam Notes and return to the Exam Room.
- To activate the Clean Room task, click on the **Waste Receptacles**.

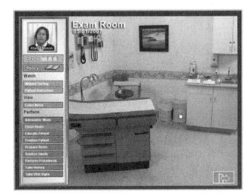

- Click to select the box next to each of the appropriate steps necessary to clean the Exam Room after Ms. Davison's visit. (Note: You can reopen the Exam Notes for reference as you make your selections.)
- Click **Finish** to return to the Exam Room.
- Click the exit arrow in the lower right corner of the screen to exit the room.
- On the Summary Menu, click on **Look at Your Performance Summary**.
- Scroll down the Performance Summary to the Clean Room section and compare your answers with those chosen by the experts.
- You may save and print the Performance Summary for your records or turn it in to your instructor. The icons for saving and printing the Performance Summary are located at the top right corner of the screen.
- Click **Close** to return to the Summary Menu.
- On the Summary Menu, click **Return to Map** and select **Yes** at the pop-up menu to return to the office map.

1. Based on your review of the Performance Summary, were there discrepancies between your steps and those of the experts? If so, what impact could these discrepancies have on patient care?

Next, you will clean the Exam Room after the physician has cared for Jesus Santo.

- From the patient list, select **Jesus Santo**.
- On the office map, click on **Exam Room**.
- Click on the **Exam Note**s file folder to read the documentation regarding Jesus Santo's visit.
- Click **Finish** to close the Exam Notes and return to the Exam Room.
- To begin cleaning the room, click on the **Waste Receptacles**.
- Use the checkboxes to select the appropriate steps necessary to clean the Exam Room after Mr. Santo's visit. (*Note:* You can reopen the Exam Notes for reference as you make your selections.)

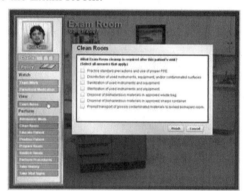

- Click **Finish** to return to the Exam Room.
- Click the exit arrow in the lower right corner of the screen to exit the room.
- On the Summary Menu, click on **Look at Your Performance Summary**.
- Scroll down the Performance Summary to the Clean Room section and compare your answers with those chosen by the experts.
- You may save and print the Performance Summary for your records or turn it in to your instructor. The icons for saving and printing the Performance Summary are located at the top right corner of the screen.
- Click **Close** to return to the Summary Menu.
- On the Summary Menu, click **Return to Map**, then click **Yes** at the pop-up menu to return to the office map.

2. Based on your review of the Performance Summary, were there discrepancies between your steps and those of the experts? If so, what impact could these discrepancies have on patient care?

Preparing the Patient and Assisting with a Routine Physical Examination

Reading Assignment: Chapter 20—The Physical Examination

Patients: Teresa Hernandez, Jean Deere

Learning Objectives:

- Identify the information needed to prepare the patient for a physical examination.
- Use the Policy Manual to determine preparation of the patient for a physical examination.
- Understand legal and ethical boundaries when preparing a patient for a physical examination.
- Choose the correct patient positioning for examination.
- Recognize the ethical role of the medical assistant when assisting with a physical examination.
- Discuss patient safety measures during a physical examination.
- Describe the importance of time efficiency when assisting the examiner.
- Understand the importance of using correct body mechanics while assisting with examinations.
- Identify the role of the medical assistant in assisting the physician with the examination and the responsibilities of the medical assistant.

Overview:

In this lesson, you will study the necessary steps in patient preparation for a routine physical examination. Teresa Hernandez is a new young patient, whereas Jean Deere is an established older adult patient. Ms. Deere wants her son James to assist in getting her ready for a physical examination. With each patient, ethical and legal issues are of concern.

Exercise 1

Writing Activity—Terms Related to Patient Examinations

 10 minutes

In the following questions, fill in the blanks with the correct terms. Use your textbook if you need help.

1. The probable course and outcome of a patient's condition is called the

   _____.

2. A physical or behavioral condition that increases the probability that an individual will

   develop a certain disease or condition is called a _____ _____.

3. A(n) _____ illness is one that has a rapid onset of symptoms, and a(n)

   _____ illness is characterized by symptoms that persist for longer than
   3 months.

4. The tests that involve the analysis and study of specimens obtained from a patient and assist

   the physician with diagnosis and treatment are _____ tests.

5. A _____ _____ is an intermediate step in the determination of

   the _____ diagnosis.

Exercise 2

Online Activity—Preparing an Established Patient for Physical Examination

 20 minutes

- Sign in to Mountain View Clinic.
- From the patient list, select **Jean Deere**.
- On the office map, click on **Exam Room**.
- Under the Watch heading, click on **Patient Assessment** and watch the video.
- Click the **X** in the upper right corner to close the video and return to the Exam Room.
- Click on **Policy** to open the office Policy Manual.
- Select **Policy Manual**, type "standing orders" in the search bar, and click on the magnifying glass.
- Read the section of the Policy Manual regarding Standing Orders.
- Click **Close Manual** to return to the Exam Room.
- Answer the following questions using the information you have just reviewed, as well as your critical thinking skills.

1. What clothing should be removed for Ms. Deere's physical examination?

2. What supplies should Armeeta ensure are available on the table to assist Ms. Deere's son James in preparing his mother for examination?

3. Armeeta has allowed Ms. Deere's son to assist with disrobing. Was that appropriate? Why or why not?

4. When would it not be appropriate or ethical to allow or suggest that a family member help disrobe a patient?

5. Why is it important for Armeeta to offer to help Ms. Deere onto the table?

6. If Armeeta had to assist with lifting Ms. Deere, which muscle groups should she use—those of the back or the large muscles of the arms and legs?

7. For safety reasons, when should Ms. Deere be positioned on the examination table?

8. Is it acceptable to leave the room when a patient who is older, confused, or debilitated is on the examination table? Why or why not?

9. What position would be appropriate for placing Ms. Deere on the exam table?

 • Click the exit arrow in the lower right corner of the screen to exit the room.

• On the Summary Menu, click **Return to Map** and select **Yes** at the pop-up menu to return to the office map.

Exercise 3

 ### Online Activity—Preparing a Young Adult and Assisting with a Routine Physical Examination

 25 minutes

• From the patient list, select **Teresa Hernandez**.
• On the office map, click on **Reception**.
• Click on the **Computer** to open the appointment book.

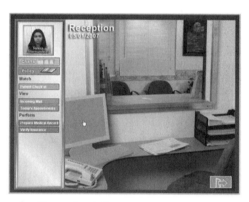

• Scroll down the appointment book to find the reason for Teresa's visit.
• Click **Finish** to close the appointment book and return to the Reception area.
• If you wish, you may also review the Standing Orders section of the Policy Manual again before answering the following questions.

1. A patient's status and the reason for an appointment will affect the preparations needed for a physical examination. What is the reason for Teresa's appointment? What is her status as a patient at Mountain View Clinic?

 • Under the Watch heading, click on **Patient Check-In** and watch Teresa Hernandez checking in to the clinic.

2. Did you think that Kristin was professional in speaking with Teresa about correcting the forms she was asked to fill out, despite the patient's concern about her parents finding out that she had an appointment at the office?

Critical Thinking Question

3. Someone else came to stand behind Teresa while she was talking with Kristin. Why do you think he was shaking his head at the end of the video?

 • Click the **X** in the upper right corner to close the video and return to the Reception area.
- Click the exit arrow in the lower right corner of the screen to exit the room.
- On the Summary Menu, click **Return to Map** and select **Yes** at the pop-up menu to return to the office map.
- On the office map, click on **Exam Room**.
- Under the Watch heading, click on **Ethical Boundaries** and watch the video.

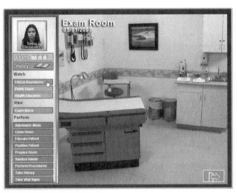

4. What preliminary steps must the clinical medical assistant complete before a physical examination is performed?

5. What clothing should Teresa remove for her examination?

6. Teresa appears to be very nervous and uneasy about discussing her chief complaint. What do you think of the way that Armeeta, the medical assistant, handled the situation?

Critical Thinking Question

7. Because of the privacy issues surrounding contraception, especially with a teenage patient, Armeeta was faced with ethical and confidentiality boundaries in preparing Teresa to talk with the physician. Do you think that Armeeta provided the guidance needed to place Teresa more at ease? Explain your answer.

8. Would it have been appropriate for Armeeta to tell Teresa that what is said in the office is confidential? Why or why not?

9. Armeeta explained to Teresa to disrobe completely and to put on the gown, but can you identify any important information that she did not include in her instructions?

→ • Click the **X** in the upper right corner to close the video and return to the Exam Room.
  • Under the Watch heading, click on **Pelvic Exam** and watch the video.

10. In the video, what are the ways that Armeeta assists Dr. Hayler? Select all that apply.

   _____ Passes the instruments

   _____ Takes the instruments after use

   _____ Waits for Dr. Hayler to ask for the instruments

   _____ Is prepared to give Dr. Hayler needed supplies promptly

   _____ Explains the procedure and the need for infection control

_____   Disposes of Dr. Hayler's disposable equipment

_____   Asks Dr. Hayler to dispose of equipment

_____   Has prepared the tray and passes all supplies on the tray for use

_____   Has the supplies prepared that might be used for a pelvic examination

_____   Accepts a specimen for laboratory testing

_____   Prepares the label for specimen transport

_____   Has the gooseneck lamp adjusted for proper lighting of the area being examined

_____   Has the patient in the proper position for a pelvic examination

11. How did Armeeta provide safety measures for Teresa?

12. What could Armeeta have asked Teresa to do before helping her sit up.

13. Why is it important for Armeeta to have all supplies and equipment available for the physician and to hand these efficiently to the physician without his asking?

14. Teresa is in the _____ position.

→ • Click the **X** in the upper right corner to close the video and return to the Exam Room.
   • Click the exit arrow in the lower right corner of the screen to exit the room.
   • On the Summary Menu, click **Return to Map** and select **Yes** at the pop-up menu to return to the office map.

Exercise 4

Writing Activity—Appropriate Body Mechanics

10 minutes

Answer the following questions regarding the use of proper body mechanics while assisting with patient examinations.

1. If you are reaching for an object, you should avoid twisting and turning and instead move your feet to face the object. What is the purpose of doing this?

2. Identify the benefits of using proper body mechanics.

3. To avoid straining the back, do not reach for something that is farther than _____ to

   _____ inches away.

4. If possible, it is better to push, pull, or slide an object rather than _____ it.

5. When standing, the feet should be in what position?

6. When sitting, what can you do to support the lower back?

7. When lifting an object, how should you bend—from the waist or from the knees?

10

Measuring Height and Weight

Reading Assignment: Chapter 20—The Physical Examination
- Measuring Weight and Height

Patients: Shaunti Begay, Jean Deere

Learning Objectives:

- Understand the correct method to use for measuring height on a teenager or an adult.
- Understand the correct method to use for measuring weight on a teenager or an adult.
- Convert height from inches to feet and inches.
- Convert height and weight from metric to English measurements.
- Convert height and weight from English to metric measurements.
- State the importance of measuring height and weight on each office visit.

Overview:

In this lesson you will view several videos regarding the correct method for measuring height and weight on a teenager and the weight of an adult. You will demonstrate how to convert a patient's height from inches to feet and inches for documentation. You will also perform conversions between metric and English measurements. One of the patients, Jean Deere, is confused. You will observe the handling of this patient and critique the actions of the medical assistant. You will also observe how a medical assistant handles a parent's negative remarks regarding her daughter's weight.

Exercise 1

Online Activity—Measuring Height

 30 minutes

- Sign in to Mountain View Clinic.
- From the patient list, select **Shaunti Begay**.
- On the office map, click on **Exam Room**.
- Under the Watch heading, click on **Health Promotion** and watch the video.

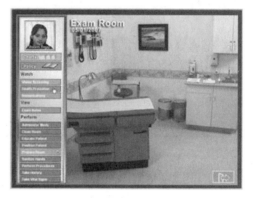

- Stop the video at the first fade-out by clicking the pause button in the lower left corner of the video screen.

1. Why should Shaunti remove her shoes before her height and weight are measured?

2. Why is measuring a child's height at each office visit important through adolescence?

Critical Thinking Question

3. Shaunti is wearing socks. If she were not wearing socks, what would have been the appropriate action by the medical assistant to ensure infection control principles before Shaunti stepped onto the scale?

4. What is the correct angle of the head bar when measuring height?

5. The height measurements on medical scales are marked in _____-inch increments.

6. The medical assistant stated that Shaunti is 5 feet 2 inches tall, which would be _____ inches.

7. How do you think Shaunti felt about her mother's comment regarding her weight?

8. In your opinion, was the medical assistant's response appropriate, or should she have dismissed the mother's comment about Shaunti's "baby fat."

- Click the **X** in the upper right corner to close the video and return to the Exam Room.
- Click the exit arrow in the lower right corner of the screen to exit the room.
- On the Summary Menu, click **Return to Map** and select **Yes** at the pop-up menu to return to the office map.

Exercise 2

Online Activity—Measuring Weight

30 minutes

1. How is quality control performed on scales?

2. What weight calibration marking is used on most standing scales found in medical offices?

- From the patient list, select **Jean Deere**.
- On the office map, click on **Exam Room**.
- Under the Watch heading, click on **Patient Assessment** and watch the video.

3. Did the medical assistant appropriately handle Ms. Deere to obtain an accurate measurement of the patient's weight?

4. The medical assistant offered to help Ms. Deere to the scales. Why would this be so important with this patient?

5. Note the placement of the walker over the scales. Why is this important to help in supporting Ms. Deere? When a walker is used in this way, what observations must the medical assistant make to ensure an accurate reading?

6. Ms. Deere is confused, and her son thinks she might have early Alzheimer disease. Do you think that the medical assistant was professional and appropriate in her handling of the patient? Explain your answer. Was it appropriate for Ms. Deere's son to be with her during the weight measurement? Why or why not?

→ • Click the **X** in the upper right corner to close the video and return to the Exam Room.

• Click on **Charts** to open Jean Deere's medical record.

• Click on the **Patient Medical Information** tab and select **1-Progress Notes** from the drop-down menu.

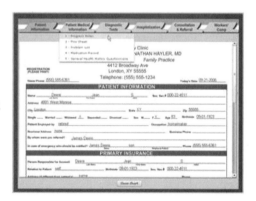

7. Based on the Progress Notes, what was Ms. Deere's weight on her last visit on 9-21-06?

8. Ms. Deere's weight on this visit is 120 pounds. Do you see a reason for the medical assistant to ask questions about her eating habits while taking the health history? Explain your answer.

 • When finished, click **Close Chart** to return to the Exam Room.
• Click on **Policy** to open the office Policy Manual.
• Select **Policy Manual** and type "standing orders" in the search bar; then click on the magnifying glass.
• Read the Standing Orders section of the Policy Manual.

9. Did the medical assistants follow the correct protocol for Shaunti Begay and Jean Deere, according to what you read in the Policy Manual? Explain your answer.

Critical Thinking Question

10. If a patient prefers not to be weighed but the protocol of the office is that all patients be weighed, what would be the best way for the medical assistant to proceed?

11. What safety steps does the medical assistant need to take with all patients when measuring weight?

 • Click **Close Manual** to return to the Exam Room.
• Click the exit arrow in the lower right corner of the screen to exit the room.
• On the Summary Menu, click **Return to Map** and select **Yes** at the pop-up menu to return to the office map or click Exit the Program.

Exercise 3

Writing Activity—Conversions for Mensuration

15 minutes

Use the formulas provided below to calculate answers to the questions in this exercise.

- Weight conversion of kilograms to pounds: Multiply kilograms by 2.2 (1 kg = 2.2 lb).
- Weight conversion of pounds to kilograms: Divide kilograms by 2.2 (2.2 lb = 1 kg).
- Height conversion of inches to feet and inches: Divide the total number of inches by 12; then express the remainder as inches (12 in = 1 ft).
- Height conversion of inches to centimeters: Multiply inches by 2.5 (1 in = 2.5 cm).
- Height conversion of centimeters to inches: Divide centimeters by 2.5 (2.5 cm = 1 in).

1. Joan Neiman weighs 64 kilograms. What is her weight in pounds?

2. Shaunti Begay is 5 feet 2 inches tall. What is her height in centimeters?

3. Jean Deere weighs 120 pounds. What is her weight in kilograms?

4. Sara McHugh is 68 inches tall. What is her height in feet and inches?

5. Isaiah Franklin is 185 centimeters tall. What is his height in inches? In feet and inches?

Eye and Ear Assessment

👓 **Reading Assignment:** Chapter 21—Eye and Ear Assessment and Procedures

Patients: Shaunti Begay, Jean Deere

Learning Objectives:

- Identify terms and abbreviations associated with eye and ear assessment.
- Differentiate the skills and responsibilities of an ophthalmologist, optometrist, and optician.
- Explain the significance of the top and bottom numbers next to each line of letters on the Snellen Eye Chart.
- Identify distractions in the office that may affect vision screening test.
- Identify the test used to assess color vision.
- Understand the difference in conductive and sensorineural hearing loss.
- Differentiate the ways in which hearing acuity can be tested.

Overview:

In this lesson you will learn important terms and abbreviations associated with eye and ear assessment. Shaunti Begay is a teenage patient who is having her vision screened while her mother stands close by. Jean Deere is an older adult patient who is having difficulty hearing; the physician will perform hearing tests on Ms. Deere. You will be asked to identify different types of hearing tests that can be performed to assess hearing.

Exercise 1

 Writing Activity—Eye and Ear Terminology and Abbreviations

10 minutes

1. Match each term or abbreviation with its definition.

Term/Abbreviation	Definition
_____ Hyperopia	a. Both ears
_____ Myopia	b. Right ear
_____ Astigmatism	c. Used to test color vision
_____ Presbyopia	d. Nearsighted vision
_____ OU	e. Farsighted vision
_____ AD	f. Refractive error; causes distortion and blurred vision
_____ AU	g. Physician who specializes in diagnosing and treating diseases and disorders of the eye
_____ Optometrist	
_____ OD	h. Licensed primary health care provider who has expertise in measuring visual acuity and prescribing corrective lenses
_____ Optician	
_____ AS	i. Professional who interprets and fills prescriptions for eyeglasses and contact lenses
_____ Ishihara test	j. Left ear
_____ Ophthalmologist	
_____ OS	k. Decreased ability to focus clearly on close objects
_____ Cerumen	l. Left eye
	m. Right eye
	n. Both eyes
	o. Earwax

Exercise 2

 CD-ROM Activity—The Eye Exam

🕐 15 minutes

- Sign in to Mountain View Clinic.
- From the patient list, select **Shaunti Begay**.

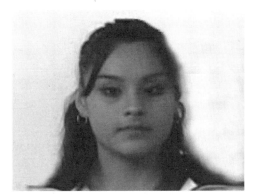

- On the office map, click on **Exam Room**.

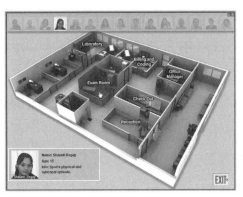

- Under the Watch heading, select **Vision Screening** to view the video.
- Click **Close** to return to the Exam Room.

1. The test Lisa is about to administer to Shaunti will assess her _____.

2. Lisa instructs Shaunti to cover one eye with the _____.

3. Lisa also shows Shaunti what she will need to read for this screening. The tool shown in the video used to measure distance vision is called the _____.

4. Shaunti is told to stand on a specific spot before beginning the test. This spot should measure a distance of _____ from the chart.

5. Why does Shaunti need to cover one eye as she reads the chart?

6. Shaunti's mother is a very active participant during Shaunti's visit. In addition to speaking for Shaunti, she is also standing very close to her during the eye exam. Is this appropriate? Why or why not?

7. Identify whether the following statement is true or false.

_____ The medical assistant was professional when she asked Shaunti's mother to allow the patient to answer the questions herself.

→ • In the Exam Room, click the exit arrow and select **Return to Map**.

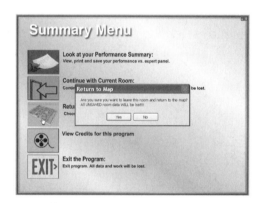

• On the office map, select **Check Out** and click to enter.

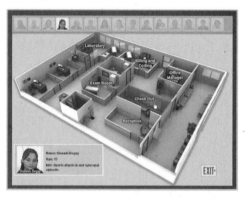

• Click on **Charts** to open Shaunti's medical record.

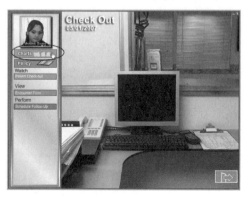

- Click on the **Patient Medical Information** tab and select **2-Progress Notes** to review the documentation of Shaunti's visit.

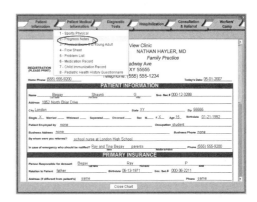

8. Scroll up to the first entry and read the results of Shaunti's vision screening. What were her results? Will Shaunti need corrective lenses?

- Click the exit arrow at the bottom right of the screen to leave the Check Out area.
- From the Summary Menu, click **Return to Map**.

9. Explain what the top and bottom numbers represent when charting vision screening results.

Exercise 3

  Online Activity—Examining the Ear

15 minutes

- From the patient list, select **Jean Deere**.
  (*Note:* If you have exited the program, sign in
  again to Mountain View Clinic and select Jean
  Deere from the patient list.)

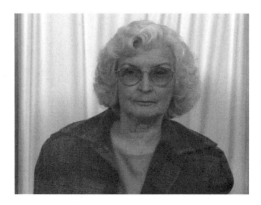

- On the office map, click on **Exam Room**.
- In the Exam Room, select **Exam Notes** to review the physician's documentation of
  Ms. Deere's exam.

1. Dr. Hayler noted Ms. Deere's exam was unremarkable, except for what finding?

2. What tests were administered to Ms. Deere relative to this finding? What were the results?

3. The _____ compares the duration of sound perception by air
   conduction with that of bone conduction.

4. The _____ helps determine whether a patient hears better in one
   ear than the other.

5. What instrument is used to perform the Rinne and Weber tests?

6. An _____ quantitatively measures hearing for the various frequencies of sound
   waves and is more specific than the Rinne and Weber tests since it provides information on
   how extensive a person's hearing loss is.

7. Based on the test results and the findings documented by Dr. Hayler, Ms. Deere has what type of hearing loss?

8. If the physician is performing the Weber hearing screen and the patient hears the sound of the tuning fork in their "good" ear, but not as well in the problem ear, what type of hearing loss would the physician document in the chart?

9. What treatment did Ms. Deere receive for this problem? What effect should this have on her symptoms?

10. What should be added to Ms. Deere's ear before irrigating it with water? Why?

Physical Agents to Promote Tissue Healing

——

/OⱭ **Reading Assignment:** Chapter 22—Physical Agents to Promote Tissue Healing

Patients: Tristan Tsosie, Janet Jones, Jose Imero

Learning Objectives:

- Identify examples of moist and dry applications of heat and cold.
- State the factors to consider when applying heat and cold.
- List the effects of local application of heat and the reasons for applying heat.
- Identify the effects of local application of cold and the reasons for applying cold.
- List factors that are taken into consideration when ambulatory aids are prescribed.

Overview:

In this lesson you will learn to distinguish between appropriate use of heat and cold application for patients, which is dependent on their complaint or symptoms. An understanding of the use of heat and cold and the physical changes each treatment brings about is important in assisting the physician with these applications in the office setting and in giving patients instructions for home application. The use of ambulatory aids is also addressed, and you will learn to recognize when their use is appropriate.

Exercise 1

Online Activity—Application of Heat and Cold

15 minutes

- Sign in to Mountain View Clinic.
- From the patient list, select **Tristan Tsosie**.

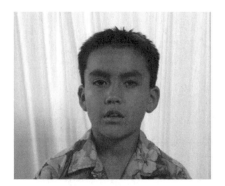

- On the office map, click on **Exam Room**.

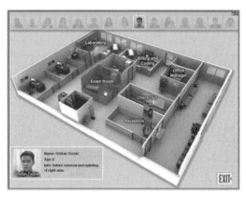

- Click on **Charts** to open Tristan's medical record.
- Under the **Consultation and Referral** tab, select **1-Consultation Notes**.
- Read the documentation for Tristan's orthopedic consultation.

1. Why was Tristan being seen by the orthopedic surgeon?

2. Scroll down through the report and read the results of Tristan's radiograph under the Imaging heading. What are the results?

3. What is the plan for Tristan documented at the end of the report?

4. What inconsistencies are present in the report?

5. The application of ice is an example of:
   a. dry cold.
   b. cold compress.
   c. moist cold.
   d. chemical cold.

6. Which of the following are valid reasons to apply ice in Tristan's case? Select all that apply.

   _____ To reduce swelling

   _____ To keep the bones in one place

   _____ To reduce pain

   _____ To decrease blood flow

   _____ To reduce the chance of infection

   _____ To keep Tristan distracted from his pain

7. Prolonged application of cold is not recommended because it has an adverse effect. Cold

   application should be removed after _____.

→ • Click **Close Chart** to return to the Exam Room.
  • Click the exit arrow and select **Return to Map**.

• On the office map, select **Janet Jones**.

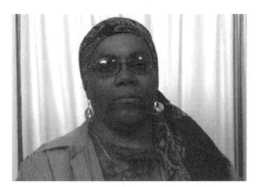

• Click on the **Exam Room** to enter.
• Click on **Exam Notes** to open the documentation of Ms. Jones' exam.

8. What is the reason for Ms. Jones' visit?

9. What type of treatment did Ms. Jones try before coming to the office to see the doctor?

10. The application of a heating pad is an example of:
    a. hot compress.
    b. moist heat.
    c. dry heat.
    d. chemical heat.

11. What are some of the benefits of applying heat in Ms. Jones' case?

12. Ms. Jones' back pain was the result of a fall, which might have strained or sprained her back. Was heat the most appropriate treatment in this case?

Critical Thinking Question

13. Why must a patient use caution with application of a heating pad?

- Click **Finish** to close the Exam Notes.
- Click the exit arrow at the bottom right of the screen.
- From the Summary Menu, click **Return to Map**.

Exercise 2

 Online Activity—Ambulatory Aids

15 minutes

- From the patient list, select **Jose Imero**. (*Note:* If you have exited the program, sign back in to Mountain View Clinic and select Jose Imero from the patient list.)

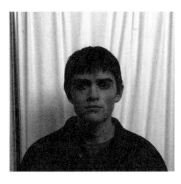

- On the office map, click on **Exam Room**.
- Inside the Exam Room, click the folder on the counter to open the **Exam Notes**.
- Read the documentation of Jose's visit.

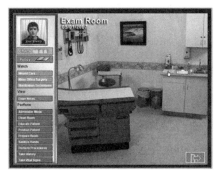

1. What is the reason for Jose's visit?

2. What is the plan for Jose's treatment?

- Click **Finish** to close the Exam Notes.
- Under the Watch heading, select **Minor Office Surgery** to view the video.
- At the end of the video, click **Close** to return to the Exam Room.

3. Charlie, the medical assistant, was fitting Jose with what type of crutches?

4. Charlie believes the crutches are too short and wants to adjust them for Jose's height. What problems could Jose encounter if the crutches are left too short?

5. After Charlie adjusts the crutches, what should he have Jose do before leaving the office? Why?

Critical Thinking Question

6. Why do you think the physician ordered crutches for Jose, instead of a cane?

The Gynecologic Examination and Prenatal Care

/ᴑᴆ **Reading Assignment:** Chapter 23—The Gynecologic Examination and Prenatal Care

Patients: Renee Anderson, Louise Parlet

Learning Objectives:

- Choose the necessary questions to ask the patient to obtain information for a thorough health history and the gynecologic and prenatal examinations.
- Understand the appropriate positions in which the patient will be placed for the gynecologic examination.
- Discuss the legal and ethical boundaries of preparing a patient for a gynecologic or prenatal examination.
- Document patient information in the medical record.
- Understand how a medical assistant should handle domestic abuse concerns ethically and professionally.
- Assess how verbal and nonverbal communications are important to assess with victims of domestic abuse.
- Read a health history form to obtain information that may indicate the patient has been abused.
- Match supplies needed during a Papanicolaou test (Pap smear) in their order of use.

Overview:

This lesson involves two patients: Louise Parlet, an established patient who is having a routine prenatal examination, and Renee Anderson, a new patient coming in for a routine gynecologic examination. Ms. Anderson is also a victim of domestic abuse.

Exercise 1

Online Activity—Assisting with a Prenatal Examination

45 minutes

- Sign in to Mountain View Clinic.
- From the patient list, select **Louise Parlet**.
- On the office map, click on **Exam Room**.
- Click on the **Exam Notes** file folder to read the documentation regarding Louise Parlet's visit.
- Click **Finish** to close the Exam Notes return to the Exam Room.
- Click on the **Supply Cabinet** to begin preparing the room for the examination.

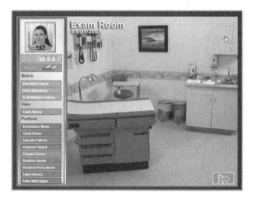

- Add the supplies needed for Louise Parlet's examination by clicking on items in the Available Supplies list and then clicking **Add Item** to confirm each choice. The items you select will appear in the Selected Supplies box. When you click on an item, a photograph of that item will appear, which can be used for reference as you review your list of supplies. (*Note:* You can reopen the Exam Notes located in the lower left corner for reference as you make your selections.)
- If you wish to remove a chosen supply, highlight the item in the Selected Supplies box and click **Remove**.
- Repeat these steps until you are satisfied you have everything you need from the list.
- Once you have made your selections, click **Finish** to return to the Exam Room.

1. Below is a list of items that will be needed for Ms. Parlet's Pap smear. Match the columns to show order in which these supplies will be used.

Order of Use	**Item**
_____ First	a. Glass slides or specimen preservative
_____ Second	b. Lubricant for rectal examination
_____ Third	c. Fixative for slides
_____ Fourth	d. Lead pencil for labeling Pap smear slides
_____ Fifth	e. Patient gown and drape
_____ Sixth	f. Laboratory requisition form and pen
_____ Seventh	g. Speculum

• Inside the Exam Room, click on the **Exam Table**.

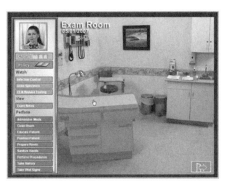

- Using the checkboxes on the screen, click to select all positions in which the patient will be placed during her examination.
- Click **Finish** to return to the Exam Room.
- Now click on the **Medical Record** clipboard to begin taking the patient's history.
- Click on the **Ask** buttons to view Louise Parlet's answers to the questions regarding her medical history.
- Record the information in the patient's medical record by keying it in the box under "Document all findings below." Enter your name after your documentation, as requested by your instructor.
- At the bottom of the page, click **Next** to view additional questions and responses related to the patient's history.
- If you think any of these additional questions need to be asked, click the corresponding checkbox for each question you want to ask.
- If requested by your instructor, print the information by clicking on **Print** at the bottom of the screen.
- Click **Finish** to close the Take History window and answer **Yes** at the pop-up window to return to the Exam Room.

2. What information is important to obtain before a prenatal examination?

3. What information did Ms. Parlet provide that might indicate that she is pregnant?

4. How many times has Ms. Parlet conceived, and what was the outcome? (*Hint:* Go back to the Exam Notes if needed. You may also open Ms. Parlet's chart and choose **5-General Health History Questionnaire** under the **Patient Medical Information** tab.)

Critical Thinking Question

5. Why might a patient who has previously had a spontaneous abortion be "afraid" of complications of pregnancy and telephone the office with questions more frequently than other patients who are pregnant?

Critical Thinking Question

6. What are ways the medical assistant can alleviate apprehension and provide emotional support to these patients?

7. List the positions that will be used for Mr. Parlet's examination in the order in which she will use them.

(1)

(2)

(3)

8. Explain the use of each of the positions listed in the previous question.

→ • Click on the **Mayo Tray** in the Exam Room to select the procedures to be performed on Louise Parlet during her examination.

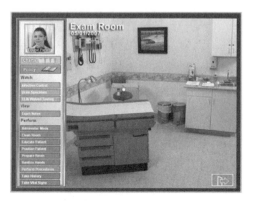

- Click on **Exam Notes** to review which procedures will be performed and to determine how many weeks Louise Parlet is pregnant.
- Click on **Finish** to return to the Perform Procedures window.
- Use the checkboxes to select the procedures that should be performed during Ms. Parlet's visit.
- Click **Finish** to return to the Exam Room.

9. Which procedures were accomplished by the medical assistant? Why were these needed for the prenatal examination?

10. According to Dr. Hayler's documentation, Ms. Parlet is _____ weeks pregnant.

11. Dr. Hayler has referred Ms. Parlet to an obstetrician to continue her prenatal care. If no problems are associated with this pregnancy, how frequently can Ms. Parlet expect to visit her obstetrician?

- Click the exit arrow in the lower right corner of the screen to exit the room.
- On the Summary Menu, click on **Look at Your Performance Summary**.
- Scroll down the Performance Summary to the sections for the task you just performed: Position Patient, Prepare Room, Perform Procedures, and Take History. For each task, compare your answers with those chosen by the experts.
- You may save and print the Performance Summary for your records or turn it in to your instructor. The icons for saving and printing the Performance Summary are located at the top right corner of the screen.
- Click **Close** to return to the Summary Menu.
- On the Summary Menu, click **Return to Map** and select **Yes** at the pop-up menu to return to the office map.

Exercise 2

Online Activity—Assisting with a Gynecologic Examination

 30 minutes

- From the patient list, select **Renee Anderson**.
- On the office map, click on **Reception**.
- Under the Watch heading, click on **Patient Check-In** and watch Renee Anderson checking in to the clinic.

1. What nonverbal communication displayed by the patient in this video is the most important for the medical assistant to observe and respond to? Explain your answer.

2. Did the medical assistant at check-in handle the confidentiality question correctly and accurately? Explain your answer.

➡️
- Click the **X** in the upper right corner to close the video and return to the Reception area.
- Click on the **Medical Record** on the counter to begin assembling a chart for Renee Anderson's visit.
- On the pop-up window, click **Perform** next to Assemble Medical Record.
- The Patient Information tab is automatically chosen as the starting point when you access the Assemble Medical Record screen.
- Add the forms you think will be needed in the Patient Information tab by selecting them from the Forms Available list and then clicking **Add** to confirm your choices. The forms you select will appear under the corresponding tab at the bottom of the screen.

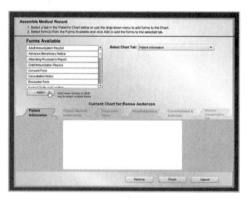

- When you have completed the Patient Information section, continue adding forms to other appropriate tabs in the patient's medical record. To select a new tab, either click on the tab on the medical record or use the drop-down menu on the right.
- If you wish to remove a chosen form, highlight the form and click **Remove** at the bottom of the screen.
- When you are satisfied that you have selected all the necessary forms and put them in the correct tab sections, click **Finish** to close the chart and return to the Reception area.

• Click the exit arrow in the lower right corner of the screen to exit the room.
  • On the Summary Menu, click **Return to Map** and select **Yes** at the pop-up menu to return to the office map.
  • On the office map, click on **Exam Room**.
  • Under the Watch heading, click on **Patient Care** and watch the video.

3. In the video, Susan states that she missed a question on the laboratory request form concerning previously abnormal Pap smears. Why is this important?

4. During the examination, what nonverbal communication did the patient provide to the medical assistant and physician that might have led to an examination for spousal abuse by the physician?

5. Do you think that Susan provided the appropriate verbal and nonverbal support for a patient whose nonverbal communication at check-in indicated an emotional problem? Explain your answer.

6. Why are the instructions for breast self-examination important to include with each gynecologic patient?

 • Click the **X** in the upper right corner to close the video and return to the Exam Room.
  • Click on **Charts** to open Renee Anderson's medical record.
  • Click on the **Patient Medical Information** tab and select **1-General Health History Questionnaire** from the drop-down menu.
  • Read the entire document. Use the arrows at the top right of the screen to turn the pages.

7. Dr. Hayler suggests that Ms. Anderson have a mammogram. Other than finding a breast lump, what reason would be appropriate for suggesting this mammogram? (*Hint:* Check the Patient Information Form in her chart for age and health history.)

8. What other information on the health history form provides a hint of spousal abuse, along with the physical findings documented on page 6 of the health history?

→ • Click **Close Chart** when finished to return to the Exam Room.
  • Under the Watch heading, click on **Communication** and watch the video.

9. When Ms. Anderson arrived for her appointment, ethical and confidential matters were discussed. What did Dr. Hayler and the medical assistant do to continue the ethical and confidential manner of the examination?

10. How do you feel about the manner that Dr. Hayler used when talking with Ms. Anderson, as well as the response of the medical assistant, Susan, to the patient's nonverbal communication?

11. What responsibilities did the medical assistant have concerning the cleaning of the room before Dr. Hayler returned to discuss treatment with Ms. Anderson?

→ • Click the **X** in the upper right corner to close the video and return to the Exam Room.
  • Click on the **Waste Receptacles**.

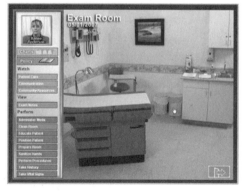

  • Use the checkboxes to select the appropriate steps necessary to clean the Exam Room after Renee Anderson's examination.
  • Click **Finish** to return to the Exam Room.

12. Indicate whether each of the following statements is true or false.

  a. _____   The date of the last menstrual period is not important to include on the laboratory requisition form for a Pap smear.

  b. _____   The medical assistant is responsible for asking the site of specimen collection during a Pap smear if this information is not provided by the physician.

  c. _____   When assisting with a pelvic examination, the medical assistant should be near the supply tray to pass needed supplies to the physician but should also be at the side of the patient to provide support and to observe nonverbal communication.

  d. _____   With a female patient and a male examiner, the medical assistant has a legal and ethical responsibility to remain in the room at all times.

- Click the exit arrow in the lower right corner of the screen to exit the room.
- On the Summary Menu, click on **Look at Your Performance Summary**.
- Scroll down the Performance Summary to the Clean Room section and compare your answers with those chosen by the experts.
- You may save and print the Performance Summary for your records or turn it in to your instructor. The icons for saving and printing the Performance Summary are located at the top right corner of the screen.
- Click **Close** to return to the Summary Menu.
- On the Summary Menu, click **Return to Map** and select **Yes** at the pop-up menu to return to the office map.

Critical Thinking Question

13. In the video, Dr. Hayler's assistant, who was present during the examination of his patient, is a woman. Why is it recommended that a female assistant, rather than Charlie, the male medical assistant, assist with the prenatal examination?

Critical Thinking Question

14. Why is important to keep the patient covered with the gown and drape as much as possible, rather than just removing the entire drape during the pelvic examination?

Critical Thinking Question

15. What legal problems could arise if the patient and physician are alone during the time the patient is disrobed during a gynecologic examination?

Critical Thinking Question

16. What should the next step be in caring for a patient who may be the victim of domestic abuse?

➝ • Under the Watch heading, click on **Community Resources** and watch the video.

17. In your opinion, did Susan give the community resource information to Ms. Anderson in a professional manner? Would you have done anything differently?

The Pediatric Examination

/OᴆᴅＯ **Reading Assignment:** Chapter 24 — The Pediatric Examination

Patient: Jade Wong

Learning Objectives:

- Describe the steps necessary in preparing a child for a pediatric examination.
- Explain the differences between obtaining mensurations in children and in adults.
- Plot height and weight on a growth chart for a child, and identify trends in percentile ranking.
- Describe the role of the medical assistant in a pediatric examination.
- Understand the importance of verbal and nonverbal communication with persons of different cultures.
- Understand the methods of parental involvement while preparing infants for physical examination.
- Read Progress Notes to obtain information about the patient's visit.

Overview:

In this lesson you will be introduced to the pediatric examination and will be expected to identify the differences in examining a pediatric patient versus an adult patient. Jade Wong's parents are of Asian descent and speak little English. During Jade's pediatric visit, the medical assistant explains the needs to the father, who acts as an interpreter. The mother is also provided information concerning immunizations for health promotion and disease prevention.

Exercise 1

Online Activity—Assisting with a Pediatric Examination

45 minutes

- Sign in to Mountain View Clinic.
- From the patient list, select **Jade Wong**.
- On the office map, click on **Reception**.
- Click on the **Medical Record** to assemble a chart for Jade Wong's visit.

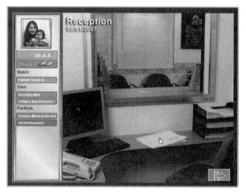

- On the pop-up window, click on the **Perform** button next to Assemble Medical Record.
- The Patient Information tab is automatically chosen as the starting point when you access the Assemble Medical Record screen.
- Add forms needed in the Patient Information tab by selecting forms from the Forms Available list and clicking **Add** to confirm your choices. The forms you select will appear under the tabs at the bottom of the screen.
- When you have completed the Patient Information section, continue adding forms to other appropriate tabs in the patient's medical record. To select a new tab, either click on the tab on the medical record or use the drop-down menu on the right.
- If you wish to remove a chosen form, highlight the form and click **Remove** at the bottom of the screen.
- When you are satisfied that you have selected all the necessary forms and put them in the correct tab sections, click **Finish** to close the chart and return to the Reception area.
- Click the exit arrow in the lower right corner of the screen to exit the room.
- On the Summary Menu, click on **Look at Your Performance Summary**.
- Scroll down the Performance Summary to the Patient Records section and compare your answers with those chosen by the experts.
- You may save and print the Performance Summary for your records or turn it in to your instructor. The icons for saving and printing the Performance Summary are located at the top right corner of the screen.
- Click **Close** to return to the Summary Menu.
- On the Summary Menu, click **Return to Map** and select **Yes** at the pop-up menu to return to the office map.
- On the office map, click on **Exam Room**.
- You will be watching a total of three videos during Jade's visit. As you watch each video, pay close attention to see whether you notice anything on the counter or in the Exam Room that does not "belong" or should not be in the room where patient care is provided.
- Under the Watch heading, select **Well-Baby Visit** and watch the video.

1. What measurements would you expect the medical assistant to obtain on Jade for a well-baby visit, and how do these measurements differ from an adult measurement?

2. Why is it important for the medical assistant to develop a rapport with the child and with the parents when assisting with a well-child office visit?

Critical Thinking Question

3. As the medical assistant works with Jade, she is using the father as an interpreter and is allowing the mother to have an active part in the medical care through this means. Do you feel this is an important part of the care, or do you believe the medical assistant should provide care and speak only with the father? Explain your answer.

4. Why is it important to remove the infant's clothing before weighing her? Why should the diaper be removed?

Critical Thinking Question

5. What are some of the differences between preparing a 4-year-old toddler for an examination and preparing an infant for an examination?

6. What tactics may be used with older children to gain their confidence?

7. What roles do verbal communication and nonverbal communication play in a pediatric examination?

 • Click the **X** in the upper right corner to close the video and return to the Exam Room.

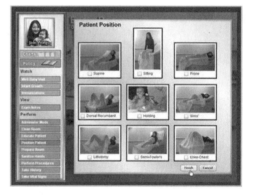

- Click on the **Exam Table**.
- Use the checkboxes to select all positions in which the patient will be placed during her examination.

- Click **Finish** to return to the Exam Room.
- Under the Watch heading, click on Infant Growth and watch the video.
- Click the **X** in the upper right corner to close the video and return to the Exam Room.
- Under the Watch heading, click on **Immunizations** and watch the video.
- Click the **X** in the upper right corner to close the video and return to the Exam Room.
- Click the exit arrow in the lower right corner of the screen to exit the room.
- On the Summary Menu, click on **Look at Your Performance Summary**.
- Scroll down the Performance Summary to the Position Patient section and compare your answers with those chosen by the experts.
- Click **Close** to return to the Summary Menu.
- On the Summary Menu, click **Return to Map** and select **Yes** at the pop-up menu to return to the office map.
- On the office map, click on **Billing and Coding**.
- Click on **Charts** to open Jade Wong's medical record.

• Click on the **Patient Medical Information** tab and select **6-Newborn Health Summary** from the drop-down menu.

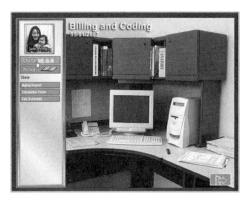

8. Record Jade's birth weight and length and her head circumference from the medical history in the Newborn Health Summary.

• Click on the **Patient Medical Information** tab and select **1-Progress Notes** from the drop-down menu.

9. What measurements were recorded from today's visit?

• Look again the Progress Notes and read the chief complaint documented for today's visit.

10. As you watched the videos of Jade's visit to the medical office, what role did the clinical medical assistant play throughout the visit?

11. Did you notice anything in the Exam Room that should not have been in the room where patient care is provided?

12. Why is the chief complaint in quotation marks?

13. Indicate whether each of the following statements is true or false.

a. _____ The growth charts are the same for both genders and for all ages.

b. _____ A well-baby visit is usually scheduled every 2 months for the first 6 months to ensure that the child receives the needed immunizations on schedule.

c. _____ After the age 6 months, the well-baby visits are scheduled every 3 months until age 18 months.

d. _____ After 2 years of age, well-child visits are scheduled every 2 years.

e. _____ The medical assistant should obtain information about the motor and cognitive development of the child at each visit.

f. _____ If a child is seen for a sick-child visit between well-baby visits, the child does not need to have weight and length obtained.

g. _____ When measuring the circumference of the head and chest, the measurement should be taken at the greatest circumference.

h. _____ Infant scales measure weight in pounds and ounces rather than in pounds and fractions of pounds as with adults.

i. _____ When measuring the height of an infant, the measurement should be from the heel to the crown of the head.

j. _____ When a child becomes old enough to stand on a scale, he or she will sometimes be difficult to weigh and may be afraid or have difficulty balancing without holding onto something.

k. _____ When weighing a young child who is afraid of the balance beam scales or who weighs more than the infant scale can accommodate, an alternative is to weigh the mother and child together on an adult scale and then weigh the mother alone. After obtaining the two weights, you can determine the weight of the child by subtracting the mother's weight from the combined weight of the two.

→ • Click **Close Chart** when finished to return to the Billing and Coding area.
 • Click the exit arrow in the lower right corner of the screen to exit the room.
 • On the Summary Menu, click **Return to Map**, then click **Yes** at the pop-up menu to return to the office map or click **Exit the Program**.

Exercise 2

Writing Activity—Plotting a Growth Chart and Recognizing Trends in Percentiles

20 minutes

1. Plot the growth chart below for Kaitlynn Griffin, using the following measurements:

   - 3 months: 22¾ inches, 11 pounds
   - 6 months: 26 inches, 14 pounds 8 ounces
   - 9 months: 27½ inches, 16 pounds 4 ounces
   - 13 months: 30½ inches, 19 pounds
   - 16 months: 31½ inches, 20 pounds 8 ounces
   - 24 months: 34¾ inches, 27 pounds

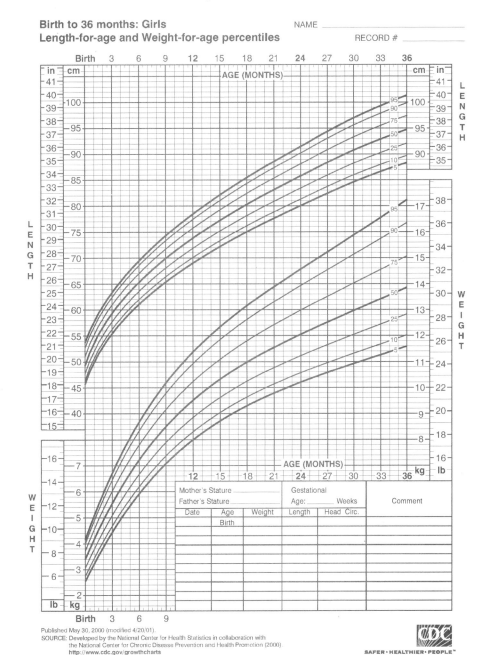

Birth to 36 months: Girls
Length-for-age and Weight-for-age percentiles

NAME _____

RECORD # _____

Published May 30, 2000 (modified 4/20/01).
SOURCE: Developed by the National Center for Health Statistics in collaboration with
the National Center for Chronic Disease Prevention and Health Promotion (2000).
http://www.cdc.gov/growthcharts

2. Compare Kaitlynn's growth percentiles. What trend do you see regarding her length?

3. What trend did you see in her weight gain?

15

Assisting with Minor Office Surgery

👓 **Reading Assignment:** Chapter 25—Minor Office Surgery

Patients: Jose Imero, Tristan Tsosie

Learning Objectives:

- Identify instruments by their use or function.
- Understand the importance of good communication skills when preparing the patient for suture removal.
- Describe the importance of infection control and sterile aseptic technique with minor surgery.
- Understand appropriate disposal of biohazardous materials when performing wound care.
- Identify instructions given to the patient during minor office surgery regarding the care of the wound and returning to the office for suture removal.
- Discuss the need for patient education after suturing a laceration and after removing sutures.
- Document chart entries pertaining to minor office surgery and suture removal.
- Apply critical thinking skills in regard to patient education related to minor office surgery.

Overview:

This lesson focuses on the medical assistant's role in assisting the physician with minor office surgery. You will observe and evaluate the medical assistant's preparation of patient Jose Imero for suturing of lacerations. Another patient, Tristan Tsosie, has a previously sutured laceration that needs suture removal. The necessary steps for this procedure will be shown and evaluated.

Exercise 1

Online Activity—Assisting with Minor Office Surgery

 45 minutes

- Sign in to Mountain View Clinic.
- From the patient list, select **Jose Imero**.
- On the office map, click on **Exam Room**.
- Begin taking the patient's history by clicking on the **Medical Record** clipboard.

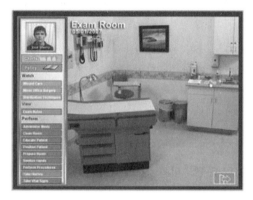

- Click on the **Ask** buttons to view Jose Imero's answers to questions regarding his medical history.
- Record the information in the patient's medical record in the box under "Document all findings below." Enter your name after your documentation, as requested by your instructor.
- At the bottom of the page, click **Next** to view additional questions and responses related to Jose Imero's history.
- Use the checkboxes to select any other question you think you should ask Jose Imero.
- If requested by your instructor, print the information by clicking on **Print** at the bottom of the screen.
- Click **Finish** to close the Take History window and answer **Yes** at the pop-up window to return to the Exam Room.
- Now click on the **Vital Signs Wall Unit**.
- Click **Take Blood Pressure**. Jose Imero's blood pressure reading will appear in the box underneath.
- Repeat this step for all vital signs.
- Record the readings in the appropriate boxes at the bottom of the screen.
- If any of the patient's results are abnormal, select the box that says, "Check if physician needs to be notified of abnormality."
- Click **Finish** to return to the Exam Room.
- Next, click on the **Exam Notes** file folder to read the documentation regarding Jose's visit. Note the procedures he is scheduled to have performed during his examination and the instructions you will need to give the patient before he leaves.

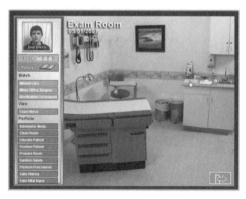

- Click **Finish** to close the Exam Notes and return to the Exam Room.
- To begin preparing the room for Jose's visit, click on the **Supply Cabinet**.
- From the list of Available Supplies, click on **Wound Care** and review the contents on the tray in the photograph.

1. Listed below are the supplies provided for wound care as shown in the photograph on your screen. Briefly explain why you think each supply is needed.

   Sterile water or saline

   Surgical soap

   Gauze pads

   Gloves

   Antiseptic swabs

➤ • From the list of Available Supplies, click on **Surgical Supply Tray** and review the contents on the tray in the photograph.

2. What disposable supplies are on the supply tray that will be needed for the suturing of Jose's foot? (*Note:* You can check your answers when you watch the video later in this exercise.)

   a.

   b.

   c.

   d.

   e.

   f.

   g.

- From the list of Available Supplies, click on **Surgical Instrument Tray** and review the contents on the tray in the photograph.
- The instrument tray contains hemostats, a needle holder, suture materials, a scalpel, and thumb forceps.

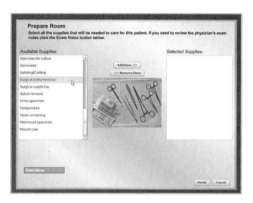

3. In the upcoming video, Dr. Hayler will specifically state that he is going to probe Jose's wound for possible foreign objects. Based on that knowledge, what sterile materials, necessary for preparing to suture a laceration, are missing from the surgical instrument tray in the photograph on your screen?

4. Match each of the following surgical instruments to its use or description.

Instrument	Use or Description
_____ Scalpel	a. Used to find foreign objects in a wound
_____ Forceps	b. Used for grasping, squeezing, and holding tissue or an item such as sterile gauze
_____ Operating scissors	c. Used to open orifices
_____ Hemostats	
_____ Needle holders	d. Instrument with straight delicate blades for cutting through tissue
_____ Retractors	e. Small surgical knife used to cut through tissue
_____ Speculum	f. Used to pull back tissue and skin
_____ Suture scissors	g. Forceps-like instrument used to hold curved needles
_____ Probe	h. Used to clamp blood vessels and to hold tissue
_____ Splinter forceps	i. Instrument with straight sharp points for removing foreign objects from wounds
	j. Used to cut sutures

- Add any supplies needed to the surgical tray for Jose Imero's examination by clicking on the supply from the Available Supplies list and clicking **Add Item** to confirm your choice. The items you select will appear in the Selected Supplies box. When you click on an item, a photograph of that item will appear, which can be used for reference as you review your list of supplies. (*Note:* You can reopen the **Exam Notes** located in the lower left corner for reference as you make your selections.)

• If you wish to remove a chosen supply, highlight the supply in the Selected Supplies box and click **Remove**.
• Repeat these steps until you are satisfied you have everything you need from the list.
• Once you have finished making your selections, click **Finish** to return to the Exam Room.
• Under the Watch heading, click on **Wound Care** and watch the video.

5. Why do you think the red bag was taped onto the Mayo stand?

6. Why did Charlie place a protective sheet under Jose's foot?

 • Click the **X** in the upper right corner to close the video and return to the Exam Room.
• Under the Watch heading, click on **Minor Office Surgery** and watch the video.
• While viewing this video, watch for a distinct break in sterile technique.

7. What is the break in sterile technique that Charlie allows to happen?

8. Why was it important for Charlie to pass the suture material around the surgical tray?

9. Using your critical thinking skills and your knowledge from the textbook chapter, indicate whether each one of the following statements is true or false.

a. _____ The medical assistant is responsible for supplying a light source when assisting with minor surgery.

b. _____ When setting a sterile field, the entire area is considered sterile.

c. _____ When preparing a tray for suturing during minor surgery, time efficiency would best be served by placing the instruments in the order of their use.

d. _____ The medical assistant should pay close attention as the surgery is being performed so that he or she can anticipate when the physician will need assistance.

e. _____ Once a minor surgery suture tray has been set, the medical assistant cannot add instruments or supplies to the tray.

f. _____ Surgical scissors may have sharp blades, blunt blades, or a combination of the two.

g. _____ When assisting with minor surgery, the medical assistant must always use sterile gloves.

h. _____ The technique used to apply sterile gloves differs from the technique used to apply nonsterile gloves.

i. _____ Selection of suture material depends on the site, length, and depth of the wound.

j. _____ When you open a sterile pack, the flap toward you should be opened first.

k. _____ A physician's choice for suture material is always the same for each wound.

l. _____ Suture material comes in absorbable and nonabsorbable types.

m. _____ Absorbable suture material is usually used for subcutaneous tissue, fascia, intestines, bladder, and peritoneum.

n. _____ Nonabsorbable sutures may be removed and are generally used for suturing skin.

o. _____ Suture material comes in varying sizes, lengths, and absorbability.

p. _____ Skin may be closed with staples and adhesive skin closures.

10. What instructions did Dr. Hayler give Jose as he was suturing his laceration?

11. Why did Dr. Hayler tell Jose to use the crutches?

Critical Thinking Question

12. Discuss some of the other reasons patients must be given instructions when they have had an area sutured.

13. What other measure did Dr. Hayler take to prevent Jose from getting an infection? (*Hint:* You may refer to the Exam Notes in the Exam Room.)

14. What other instructions were given to the patient, according to the Exam Notes?

→ • Click the **X** in the upper right corner to close the video and return to the Exam Room.
• Click the exit arrow in the lower right corner of the screen to exit the Exam Room.
• On the Summary Menu, click on **Look at Your Performance Summary**.
• Scroll down the Performance Summary to the sections pertaining to the tasks you performed during this exercise: Prepare Room, Take History, and Take Vital Signs. For each section, compare your answers with those chosen by the experts.
• You may save and print the Performance Summary for your records or turn it in to your instructor. The icons for saving and printing the Performance Summary are located at the top right corner of the screen.
• Click **Close** to return to the Summary Menu.
• On the Summary Menu, click **Return to Map** and select **Yes** at the pop-up menu to return to the office map.

Exercise 2

Online Activity—Assisting with Suture Removal

20 minutes

- From the patient list, select **Tristan Tsosie**.
- On the office map, click on **Exam Room**.
- Under the Watch heading, click on **Wound Care** and watch the video.

1. Tristan had a wound culture taken. When should the cleansing of the stitches or wound take place?

2. In the video, as the medical assistant was preparing Tristan for the removal of sutures, Tristan asked whether the procedure would hurt. Should the medical assistant have answered the question before continuing with the procedure, or was it more effective to ignore the question at that point? Explain.

Critical Thinking Question

3. Why do you think Tristan asked whether the procedure would hurt?

Critical Thinking Question

4. Would you expect most children to be as calm as Tristan was during this procedure?

• Click the **X** in the upper right corner to close the video and return to the Exam Room.
- Click on the **Supply Cabinet**.
- From the list of Available Supplies, click on **Suture Removal** and review the contents on the tray in the photograph on your screen.

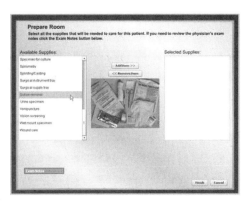

- The tray contains surgical soap, nonsterile gloves, sterile gloves, bandaging materials, gauze pads, suture-removing scissors, forceps, and a protective drape.

5. When removing sutures, what supplies should be sterile and what supplies can be aseptically clean?

6. Indicate whether each one of the following statements is true or false. Remember to use your critical thinking skills in addition to your knowledge from the reading assignment.

   a. _____ Before removing sutures, the medical assistant should obtain the permission of the physician.

   b. _____ If the wound appears to gape open during suture removal and the physician has stated that all sutures should be removed, the medical assistant should continue to remove the sutures.

   c. _____ When sutures are being removed, the patient should be placed in a comfortable position to prevent injury or unnecessary discomfort.

   d. _____ All sutures will be ready to be removed at the same time after injury.

   e. _____ The size and location of the wound are important factors in deciding when sutures will be removed.

   f. _____ All sutures may be removed using the same size of suture scissors and forceps.

   g. _____ When sutures are being removed, the suture should be cut as close to the skin as possible and then pulled in the opposite direction to prevent the microorganisms from passing through the skin into the wound.

   h. _____ When cleansing the area before removing sutures, the skin should be thoroughly cleansed and the exudate removed.

   i. _____ When you are removing sutures, it is not important to count the sutures you have removed, because you only need to remove the ones that you can see.

• Add the supplies needed for the patient's examination by clicking on the supply from the Available Supplies list and clicking **Add Item** to confirm your choice. The items you select will appear in the Selected Supplies box. When you click on an item, a photograph of that item will appear, which can be used for reference as you review your list of supplies. (Note: You can reopen the Exam Notes located in the lower left corner for reference as you make your selections.)

• If you wish to remove a chosen supply, highlight the supply in the Selected Supplies box and click **Remove**.

• Repeat these steps until you are satisfied you have everything you need from the list.

• Once you have made your selections, click **Finish** to return to the Exam Room.

• Now click on the **Waste Receptacles**.

• Use the checkboxes to select the appropriate steps necessary to clean the Exam Room after Tristan's examination.

• Click **Finish** to return to the Exam Room.

7. Explain the importance of patient education regarding the proper care of the wound at home after suturing and suture removal.

8. On the form below, document the removal of sutures from a clean wound on Tristan Tsosie's arm. These sutures had been inserted 6 days earlier. Be sure to document that the physician, Dr. Hayler, has observed the sutures and has told you to remove these seven sutures. In addition, document the dressing of the wound after removal and that the patient did not seem to have any problems. Use today's date for the documentation and your initials for the entry.

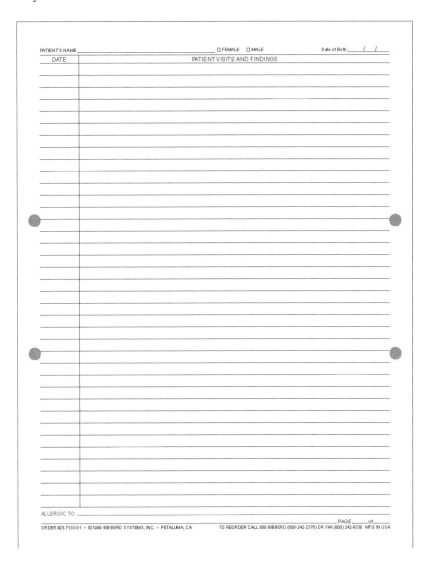

 • Click the exit arrow in the lower right corner of the screen to exit the room.

• On the Summary Menu, click on **Look at Your Performance Summary**.

• Scroll down the Performance Summary to the Clean Room section and the Prepare Room section and compare your answers with those chosen by the experts.

• You may save and print the Performance Summary for your records or turn it in to your instructor. The icons for saving and printing the Performance Summary are located at the top right corner of the screen.

• Click **Close** to return to the Summary Menu.

• On the Summary Menu, click **Return to Map**, then click **Yes** at the pop-up menu to return to the office map or click **Exit the Program**.

LESSON 16

Administration of Medication and Intravenous Therapy

Reading Assignment: Chapter 24 — The Pediatric Examination
- Pediatric Injections
- Immunizations

Chapter 26 — Administration of Medication and Intravenous Therapy
- Systems of Measurement for Medication
- Prescription
- Medication Record
- Guidelines for Preparation and Administration of Medication
- Parenteral Administration

Patients: Shaunti Begay, Jesus Santo, Jade Wong

Learning Objectives:

- Identify the correct dose (volume) of medication for a patient using the physician's order.
- Choose appropriate supplies for assisting with medication administration (based on volume ordered).
- Identify the correct supplies to use for medication administration.
- List the seven "rights" of patient medication administration.
- Identify the steps that should be taken to ensure patient safety with the administration of medications.
- Identify local resources for immunizations and for patient education.
- Correlate the importance of timing the collection of laboratory specimens with medication administration.
- Prepare a written prescription for the physician's signature using an order written in the patient's chart.
- Choose the appropriate biohazard container for the disposal of supplies used in medication administration.
- Understand the documentation and record-keeping procedures for administering medications and immunizations.
- Correctly document medication administration.

161

Overview:

This lesson presents the administration of medication based on the physician's order. You will choose syringes and volume of medication to help prepare patients for the administration of parenteral medications and immunizations. You will also complete documentation of these injections. The appropriate way to provide referrals to community resources for health maintenance and prevention is also presented.

Exercise 1

Online Activity—Administering Parenteral Medications

30 minutes

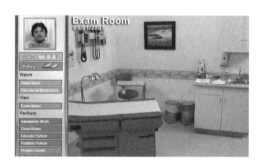

- Sign in to Mountain View Clinic.
- From the patient list, select **Jesus Santo**.
- On the office map, click on **Exam Room**.
- Click on the **Exam Notes** file folder to read the documentation regarding Jesus Santo's visit.
- Click **Finish** to close the Exam Notes and return to the Exam Room.
- Now begin to prepare the room for Mr. Santo's visit by clicking on the **Supply Cabinet**.
- Add the supplies needed for Jesus Santo's examination by clicking on the supply from the Available Supplies list and clicking **Add Item** to confirm your choice. The items you select will appear in the Selected Supplies box. When you click on an item, a photograph of that item will appear, which can be used for reference as you review your list of supplies. (*Note:* You can reopen the Exam Notes located in the lower left corner for reference as you make your selections.)
- If you wish to remove a chosen supply, highlight the supply in the Selected Supplies box and click **Remove**.
- Repeat these steps until you are satisfied you have everything you need from the list.
- Keep the Prepare Room window open as you continue with the lesson.

1. The medical assistant is asked to prepare Bicillin-LA 1,200,000 units for injection. If the medication is available as Bicillin-LA 600,000 units/mL, how many milliliters should Charlie prepare to give Mr. Santo?

2. What is the classification of Bicillin-LA? (*Hint:* Refer to Table 26-1 in the textbook if you need help.)

• From the list of Available Supplies, click on **Parenteral Injection** and review the contents on the tray in the photograph.

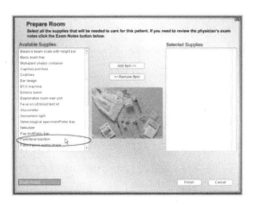

3. On the tray are four syringes: a tuberculin syringe, a 5-mL syringe, an insulin syringe, and a 3-mL syringe. Which is the correct syringe for the administration of the medication ordered?

4. Below, choose the correct syringe to use; then indicate the amount of medication that should be given to Jesus Santo by shading in the appropriate area on the syringe you selected.

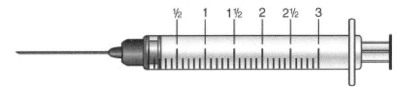

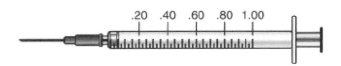

• Click **Finish** to close the Prepare Room window and return to the Exam Room.

5. After the administration of Bicillin-LA, the syringe should be disposed in which of the following containers?
   a. Regular waste container
   b. Biohazard waste container
   c. Puncture-proof biohazard waste container

6. Which container is appropriate for disposal of used supplies, other than the syringe, after the administration of Bicillin-LA?
   a. Regular waste container
   b. Biohazard waste container
   c. Puncture-proof biohazard waste container

7. On the form below, properly document the injection given to Mr. Santo using the present date and time.

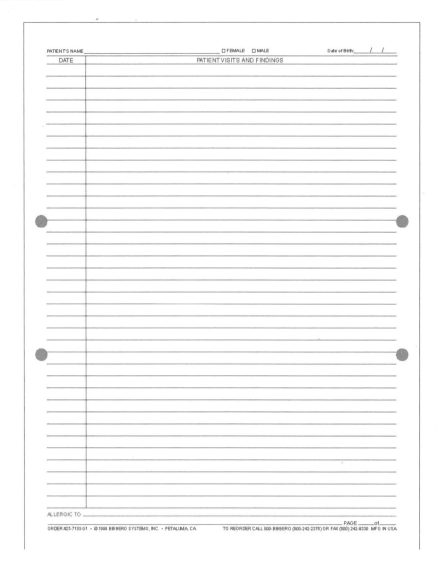

8. The Exam Notes state that the complete blood count (CBC) should be drawn before administering Bicillin-LA. Why should the CBC be drawn first and then the medication administered?

9. Why is it important for Mr. Santo to stay in the office for 20 minutes after the injection of Bicillin LA?

Critical Thinking Question

10. The physician has stated in the Exam Notes that the patient should wait for 15 to 20 minutes before leaving the office. However, Mr. Santo was brought to the medical office by his employer, Mr. Freeman. If Mr. Freeman does not want to wait, what should the medical assistant at the check-out desk do? Apply your critical thinking skills while answering this question.

11. The Exam Notes state that Mr. Santo should receive two written prescriptions. Fill out the following blank prescription forms so that they are ready for the physician's signature. For the Drug Enforcement Administration (DEA) number, use 33344888.

Mountain View Clinic
4412 Broadway Ave
London XY 55555

Phone 555-555-1234   FAX   555-555-1239

Patient Name _____ Age _____
Address _____ Date _____

℞ } Superscription

Inscription { _____

Subscription { _____

Signatura { _____

☐ Dispense as Written

Refill   NR   1   2   3   4

Signature _____
DEA # _____

Mountain View Clinic
4412 Broadway Ave
London XY 55555

Phone 555-555-1234   FAX   555-555-1239

Patient Name _____ Age _____
Address _____ Date _____

℞ } Superscription

Inscription { _____

Subscription { _____

Signatura { _____

☐ Dispense as Written

Refill   NR   1   2   3   4

Signature _____
DEA # _____

- Click the exit arrow in the lower right corner of the screen to exit the Exam Room.
- On the Summary Menu, click on **Look at Your Performance Summary**.
- Scroll down the Performance Summary to the Prepare Room section and compare your answers with those chosen by the experts.
- You may save and print the Performance Summary for your records or turn it in to your instructor. The icons for saving and printing the Performance Summary are located at the top right corner of the screen.
- Click **Close** to return to the Summary Menu.
- On the Summary Menu, click **Return to Map** and select **Yes** at the pop-up menu to return to the office map.

Exercise 2

 Online Activity—Administering and Documenting Immunizations

 30 minutes

- From the patient list, select **Shaunti Begay**.
- On the office map, click on the **Exam Room**.
- Under the Watch heading, click on **Immunizations** and watch the video.

1. What was the site of the hepatitis B immunization?

2. When is the next dose of hepatitis B due?

3. During the preparation of the hepatitis B vaccine, when should the medical assistant check the medication against the physician's order?

- Click the **X** in the upper right corner to close the video and return to the Exam Room.
- Click the exit arrow in the lower right corner of the screen to exit the room.
- On the Summary Menu, click **Return to Map** and select **Yes** at the pop-up menu to return to the office map.
- On the office map, click on **Check Out**.
- Click on **Charts** to open Shaunti Begay's medical record.

- Click on the **Patient Medical Information** tab and select **2-Progress Notes** from the drop-down menu.

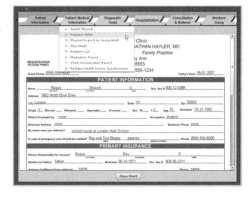

- Read the documentation regarding Shaunti Begay's immunization.

4. What volume of hepatitis B vaccine was given to Shaunti?

5. On the diagram below, shade in the appropriate area to indicate the amount of vaccine that was administered to Shaunti for the hepatitis B immunization.

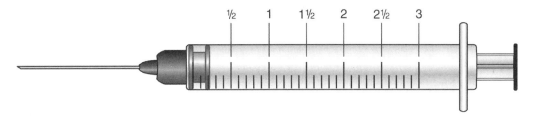

6. What is the expiration date of the hepatitis B vaccine?

7. What is a VIS? Why is this statement required for an immunization?

8. What are the seven "rights" of medication administration?

9. Why is it important to document the manufacturer of an immunizing agent, as well as the lot number and expiration date? (*Hint:* Refer to Procedure 26-4, step 15, in your textbook if you need help answering this question.)

- Click **Close Chart** when finished to return to the Check Out area.
- Click the exit arrow in the lower right corner of the screen to exit the room.
- On the Summary Menu, click **Return to Map** and select **Yes** at the pop-up menu to return to the office map.

Exercise 3

Online Activity—Immunizations as Indicated in Well-Child Visits

25 minutes

- From the patient list, select **Jade Wong**.
- On the office map, click on **Exam Room**.
- Under the Watch heading, click on **Immunizations** to view the video.

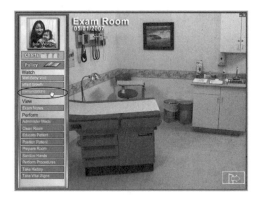

- When you are finished, click the **X** in the upper right corner to close the video and return to the Exam Room.
- Click on the **Exam Notes** file folder to read the documentation regarding Jade Wong's visit.

1. Why is it important to provide Jade's parents with information, including the VIS, concerning the immunizations their child will receive?

2. The medical assistant asked whether Jade had any problems with previous immunizations. Why is this information important before administering the immunizations at this visit?

3. What immunizations will be given to Jade? Include (spell out) the diseases against which these immunizations protect (not just the abbreviations of the immunizations).

4. The Exam Notes indicate that Jade's mother has not received the poliomyelitis (polio) vaccine. Why is the injectable polio vaccine (IPV) safer for the mother?

5. What resources are available in your community for the mother to obtain the polio vaccine if she wants to get it somewhere other than the physician's office?

→ • Click on **Finish** to close the Exam Notes and return to the Exam Room.
   • Click the exit arrow in the lower right corner of the screen to exit the room.
   • On the Summary Menu, click **Return to Map** and select **Yes** at the pop-up menu to return to the office map.
   • On the office map, click on **Check Out**.
   • Click on **Charts** to open Jade's medical record.
   • Click on the **Patient Medical Information** tab and select **1-Progress Notes** from the drop-down menu.
   • Read the documentation of Jade's examination.

6. In the Progress Notes, the medical assistant states that Jade seemed to tolerate the immunizations with no problems. Why is this documentation important?

7. What volume of Pediarix will be administered to Jade?

8. Shade the appropriate area of the syringe below to indicate the volume of Pediarix that Jade should receive.

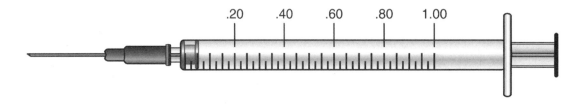

9. On the following form, document the immunizations that have been administered to Jade today, being careful to follow CDC guidelines.

Vaccine Administration Record for Children and Teens

Patient name: _____

Birthdate: _____

Chart number: _____

Before administering any vaccines, give copies of all pertinent Vaccine Information Statements (VISs) to the child's parent or legal representative and make sure he/she understands the risks and benefits of the vaccine(s). Always provide or update the patient's personal record card.

Vaccine	Type of Vaccine[1]	Date given (mo/day/yr)	Funding Source (F,S,P)[2]	Site[3]	Vaccine		Vaccine Information Statement (VIS)		Vaccinator[5] (signature or initials & title)
					Lot #	Mfr.	Date on VIS[4]	Date given[4]	
Hepatitis B[6] (e.g., HepB, Hib-HepB, DTaP-HepB-IPV) Give IM.[7]									
Diphtheria, Tetanus, Pertussis[6] (e.g., DTaP, DTaP/Hib, DTaP-HepB-IPV, DT, DTaP-IPV/Hib, Tdap, DTaP-IPV, Td) Give IM.[7]									
Haemophilus influenzae **type b**[6] (e.g., Hib, Hib-HepB, DTaP-IPV/Hib, DTaP/Hib) Give IM.[7]									
Polio[6] (e.g., IPV, DTaP-HepB-IPV, DTaP-IPV/Hib, DTaP-IPV) Give IPV SC or IM.[7] Give all others IM.[7]									
Pneumococcal (e.g., PCV7, PCV13, conjugate; PPSV23, polysaccharide) Give PCV IM.[7] Give PPSV SC or IM.[7]									
Rotavirus (RV1, RV5) Give orally (po).									
Measles, Mumps, Rubella[6] (e.g., MMR, MMRV) Give SC.[7]									
Varicella[6] (e.g., VAR, MMRV) Give SC.[7]									
Hepatitis A (HepA) Give IM.[7]									
Meningococcal (e.g., MCV4; MPSV4) Give MCV4 IM7 and MPSV4 SC.[7]									
Human papillomavirus (e.g., HPV2, HPV4) Give IM.[7]									
Influenza (e.g., TIV, inactivated; LAIV, live attenuated) Give TIV IM.[7] Give LAIV IN.[7]									
Other									

How to Complete this Record

1. Record the generic abbreviation (e.g., Tdap) or the trade name for each vaccine (see table at right).
2. Record the funding source of the vaccine given as either F (federal), S (state), or P (private).
3. Record the site where vaccine was administered as either RA (right arm), LA (left arm), RT (right thigh), LT (left thigh), or IN (intranasal).
4. Record the publication date of each VIS as well as the date the VIS is given to the patient.
5. To meet the space constraints of this form and federal requirements for documentation, a healthcare setting may want to keep a reference list of vaccinators that includes their initials and titles.
6. For combination vaccines, fill in a row for each antigen in the combination.
7. IM is the abbreviation for intramuscular; SC is the abbreviation for subcutaneous; IN is the abbreviation for intranasal.

Abbreviation	Trade Name & Manufacturer
MMR	MMRII (Merck)
VAR	Varivax (Merck)
MMRV	ProQuad (Merck)
HepA	Havrix (GlaxoSmithKline [GSK]); Vaqta (Merck)
HepA-HepB	Twinrix (GSK)
HPV2	Cervarix (GSK)
HPV4	Gardasil (Merck)
LAIV (Live attenuated influenza vaccine)	FluMist (MedImmune)
TIV (Trivalent inactivated influenza vaccine)	Afluria (CSL Biotherapies); Agriflu (Novartis); Fluarix (GSK); FluLaval (GSK); Fluvirin (Novartis); Fluzone (sanofi)
MCV4	Menactra (sanofi pasteur); Menveo (Novartis)
MPSV4	Menomune (sanofi pasteur)

Technical content reviewed by the Centers for Disease Control and Prevention, March 2011.

For additional copies, visit www.immunize.org/catg.d/p2022.pdf • Item #P2022 (3/11)

This form was created by the Immunization Action Coalition • www.immunize.org • www.vaccineinformation.org

10. Why is the use of a 1-mL syringe more appropriate for administering the medication to Jade?

 • When finished, click **Close Chart** to return to the Check Out desk.

• Under the Watch heading, click on **Patient Check-Out** and watch Jade Wong and her parents checking out of the clinic.

11. The medical assistant provides Jade's father, Mr. Wong, with information concerning child nutrition and community resources. First, she indicates that Mr. Wong and his wife are open to this help. Why is receiving implied permission, either verbally or nonverbally, important before providing this information?

12. The Progress Notes also state that Jade's mother has been referred to ESL classes. What does the abbreviation *ESL* stand for?

13. Using the Internet or a hard-copy reference source, list the local resources available for ESL education in your area.

• Click the **X** in the upper right corner to close the video and return to the Check Out area.

• Click the exit arrow in the lower right corner of the screen to exit the room.

• On the Summary Menu, click **Return to Map**, then click **Yes** at the pop-up menu to return to the office map or click **Exit the Program**.

Cardiopulmonary Procedures: Electrocardiogram

𝄢 **Reading Assignment:** Chapter 12—Circulatory System
- Heart

Chapter 27—Cardiopulmonary Procedures
- Conduction System of the Heart
- Cardiac Cycle
- Electrocardiograph Paper
- Standardization of the Electrocardiograph
- Electrocardiograph Leads
- Electrocardiographic Capabilities
- Artifacts
- Holter Monitor Electrocardiography

Patients: John R. Simmons, Shaunti Begay

Learning Objectives:

- Discuss the purpose of electrocardiography (ECG).
- Understand when Holter monitoring would be indicated.
- Describe the general anatomy of the heart.
- Identify the correct placement of leads for an ECG.
- Identify the waves, segments, and intervals that show up on an ECG representative of the cardiac cycle.
- State the need for quality control and the use of standardization marks when performing ECGs.
- Discuss the proper way to handle ECG paper.
- Describe patient preparation for an ECG.
- Identify the 12 leads found on an ECG.
- Understand what artifacts are and what can cause them.
- Discuss ways of maintaining professionalism and ethical behavior to make a patient more comfortable when performing an ECG.
- Identify modifications in lead placement if the patient has amputations, wounds, or injuries.
- Correctly document that an ECG was performed on a patient.
- Prepare written information to give to a patient about the use of a Holter monitor and event recording.

173

Overview:

In this lesson, Dr. John R. Simmons, a college professor, will have a routine ECG. You will be asked to show your knowledge of the heart and discuss the means of testing the electrical activity of the heart. Shaunti Begay has questions about the event recording that the cardiology clinic will be performing. To alleviate her fears before she sees the cardiologist, you will prepare a general information pamphlet to give Shaunti and her parents regarding the purpose of Holter monitoring and event recording.

Exercise 1

Writing Activity—Structure of the Heart and Holter Monitoring

10 minutes

1. The heart has _____ chambers. The top chambers are called

   _____, and the bottom chambers are called _____.

2. The _____ are the smaller of the four chambers.

3. The most muscular chamber of the heart is the _____ because it serves to pump

   blood to the entire _____.

4. The two large veins that bring blood back into the heart after it has circulated are the

   _____ and the _____.

5. Without any neural stimulation, the sinoatrial (SA) node rhythmically initiates impulses at

   a rate of _____ to _____ times per minute.

6. What is the purpose of having a patient wear a Holter monitor?

7. Another term for a Holter monitor is a(n) _____, which can

   be abbreviated as _____.

8. What are some of the indications for ordering a Holter monitor test?

Exercise 2

Writing Activity—Understanding the Purpose and Components of an Electrocardiogram

45 minutes

This exercise focuses on the basic understanding of the components of electrical conduction in the heart.

1. What is an electrocardiograph?

2. Describe the electrical conduction of the heart from the inception at the SA node through the electrical impulses to the fibers of the ventricles.

3. Define *cardiac cycle*.

4. What does an ECG cycle represent?

5. Label the diagram below to show the main structures of the heart.

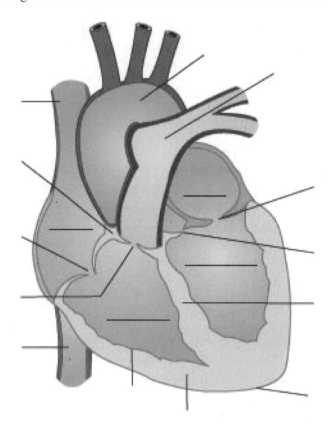

6. Label the waves, segments, and intervals on the following ECG tracing.

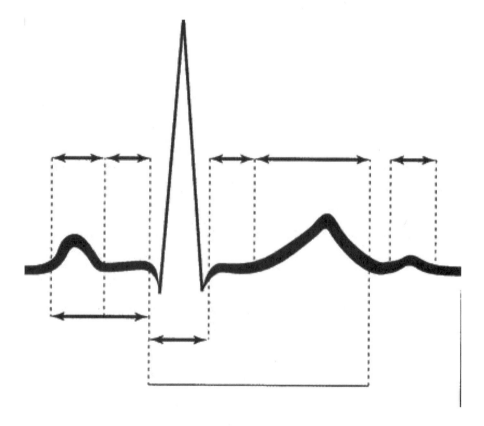

7. What does a wave in an ECG tracing indicate?

8. What does a segment on an ECG tracing indicate?

9. What does the S-T segment in an ECG tracing indicate?

10. What electrical activity of the heart is indicated by the P wave?

11. What electrical activity is indicated by the T wave?

12. What does an interval indicate on an ECG tracing?

13. What does the QRS complex indicate on an ECG tracing?

14. How does the physician use ECG paper to interpret the tracing?

15. Why is it important that the ECG tracing be handled carefully and not be allowed to smear or be folded in any way?

16. What is the purpose of the standardization mark on an ECG? How is it used?

17. List the 12 leads that are found on an ECG.

Exercise 3

 Online Activity—Preparing for the Electrocardiogram

30 minutes

1. On the diagram below, show the locations and markings of the electrodes to be placed for obtaining a 12-lead ECG.

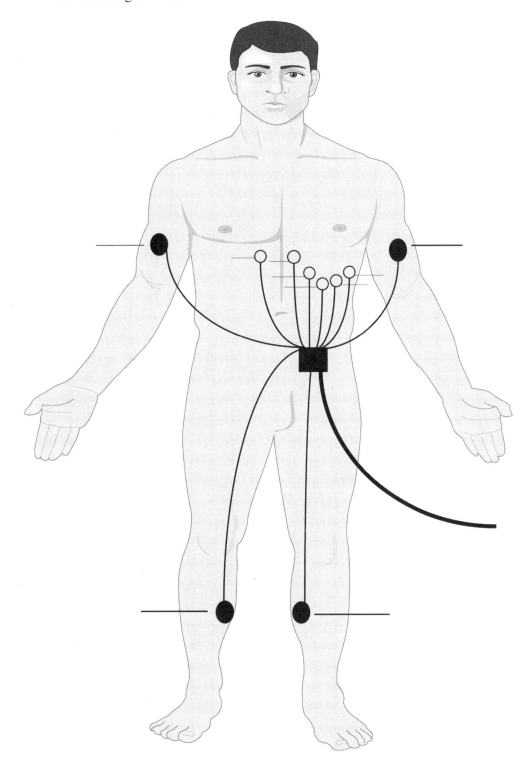

Critical Thinking Questions

Questions 2 through 5 require critical thinking. Your textbook may not include all of the answers, but these are circumstances that you may encounter as a medical assistant. If you need to refer to another source, please document the source you used.

2. If Dr. Simmons had a limb amputation or a bandage or cast on one of his extremities, how would the ECG lead be placed?

3. How should electrodes be placed on patients who have lesions, wounds, or incisions on the chest?

4. Another patient, Alice Frederick, is to have an ECG. She is obese and has pendulous breasts. How can you place the electrodes on Ms. Frederick?

5. What clothing should Ms. Frederick remove for accurate placement of the electrodes?

→ • Sign in to Mountain View Clinic.
  • From the patient list, select **John R. Simmons**.
  • On the office map, click on **Exam Room**.

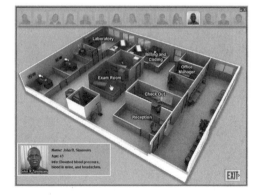

  • Under the Watch heading, click on **ECG Testing** and watch the video.
  • Stop the video at the first fade-out by clicking the pause button in the lower left corner of the video screen.

6. Describe Dr. Simmons' position on the table and how he is dressed in preparation for his ECG. Based on your observations, do you think that he has been appropriately prepared for the ECG?

Critical Thinking Question

7. Is it always necessary to have the patient remove his or her shoes and socks when performing an ECG? Why or why not?

8. Dr. Simmons asked Danielle, the medical assisting extern, whether everything was all right. He also stated that his hand was itching during the ECG. Why do you think Dr. Simmons tried to offer a reason for a problem with the ECG?

9. Imagine that you were the patient. What reaction do you think you would have if you saw such a perplexed look on the face of the medical assisting extern?

10. Danielle then stated that the recording was "fuzzy." What are fuzzy lines on the ECG called? What causes these lines?

11. What steps did Danielle take to correct this problem? What other steps could have been taken if her initial attempts had not corrected the problem?

12. Why is it important for Danielle to be sure the abnormal tracing is an artifact, rather than a dysrhythmia?

→ • Resume the video by clicking the play button in the lower left corner of the video screen.
  • As you observe the video, consider whether you think Danielle acted professionally.
  • Once again, pause the video at the next fade-out.

13. Do you think Danielle acted in a professional manner when discussing the ECG tracing with Dr. Simmons? Explain your answer.

→ • Click the play button and watch the remainder of the video.

14. Do you feel that the medical assistant correctly handled the fact that Danielle had discussed the ECG tracing with Dr. Simmons? Explain your answer.

15. On the blank Progress Notes form below, document the obtaining of the ECG on Dr. Simmons. Use today's date and time for the documentation.

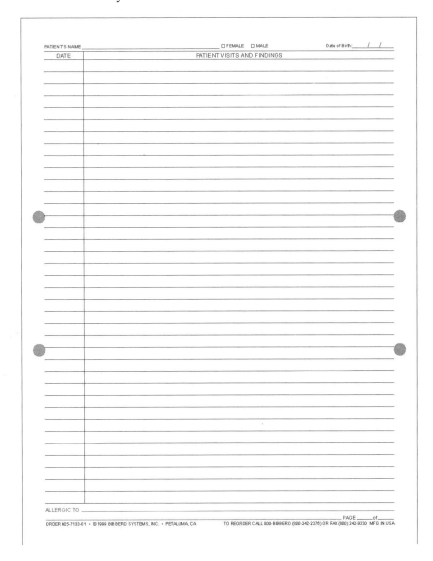

• Click the **X** in the upper right corner to close the video and return to the Exam Room.
• Click the exit arrow in the lower right corner of the screen to exit the room.
• On the Summary Menu, click **Return to Map**, then click **Yes** at the pop-up menu to return to the office map or click **Exit the Program**.

Exercise 4

 Writing Activity—Responding to a Patient's E-Mail Inquiry Concerning Cardiology Testing

 10 minutes

1. Shaunti Begay is being referred to a cardiology clinic for follow-up of her syncopal episodes and fainting. Shaunti sends an e-mail message to the office and tells you that she is "afraid" about having a Holter monitor and event testing and "worried" about her approaching appointment with the cardiologist.

   Below, compose a short informational e-mail message to send to Shaunti. (*Hint:* If you need to refer to Shaunti's Progress Notes, sign in to Mountain View Clinic and select **Shaunti Begay** as your patient. Click on the **Check Out** area and then click on **Charts**. Click on the **Patient Medical Information** tab and select **2-Progress Notes** from the drop-down menu.)

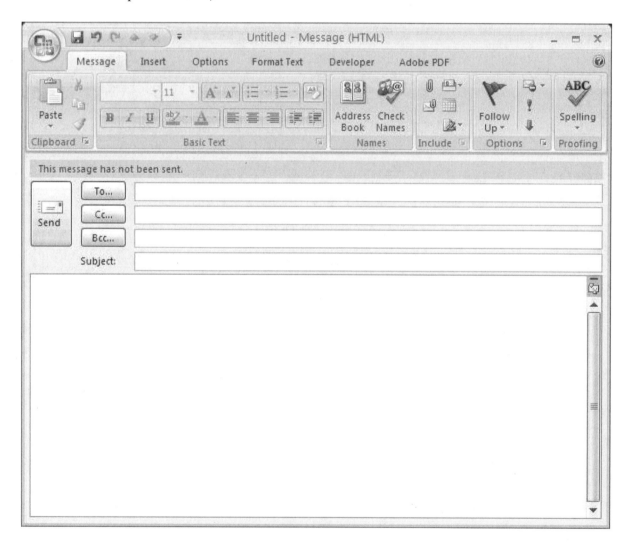

18

Respiratory Testing Procedures

/OO **Reading Assignment:** Chapter 27—Cardiopulmonary Procedures
- Pulmonary Function Test
- Peak Flow Measurement
- Home Oxygen Therapy

Patients: John R. Simmons, Hu Huang

Learning Objectives:

- Understand the purpose of pulmonary function tests.
- Be familiar with abbreviations associated with pulmonary function tests and know their definitions.
- Identify pulmonary function tests performed in the physician's office.
- Identify indications for spirometry testing.
- Distinguish among pulmonary function tests.
- Identify the necessary steps in patient preparation for respiratory testing.
- Understand the unique role of the medical assistant in spirometry testing.
- Identify possible reasons for obtaining a sputum specimen.
- Correctly document respiratory testing results in the patient's Progress Notes.
- Explain the benefits of peak flow measurements in monitoring patients who have asthma.
- Give examples of patients who may need home oxygen therapy.

Overview:

This lesson is designed to provide instruction in respiratory testing and the proper documentation of the procedure. Dr. John R. Simmons, a college professor, will have respiratory testing as part of his complete medical examination. Another patient, Hu Huang, has a suspected diagnosis of avian flu that he may have acquired during a trip to Asia. He will be providing sputum specimens for a differential diagnosis. Standard precautions will be necessary while performing the test and when discarding supplies after the testing is complete and sputum is collected. You will be asked to explain the role of peak flow monitoring in controlling asthma symptoms and give examples of patients who may need to have oxygen therapy administered in their homes.

Exercise 1

Writing Activity—Elements in Respiratory Testing

20 minutes

1. What are the purposes of pulmonary function tests?

2. Identify and briefly describe the method of pulmonary function testing that is frequently performed in the physician's office setting.

3. List at least three indications for spirometry testing.

4. Indicate whether each of the following questions pertaining to patient preparation for spirometry testing is true or false.

   a. _____ The patient should stop smoking at least 2 hours before the test is performed.

   b. _____ Clothing worn during the spirometry test should be loose, and the patient's chest area should be kept as free as possible.

   c. _____ A patient should take all of his or her medications as usual before the test.

   d. _____ The reason the patient should not eat a heavy meal 8 hours before testing is to prevent weight gain.

   e. _____ You should advise the patient not to exercise for 4 hours before the test.

5. Discuss the indications for postbronchodilator spirometry testing.

Exercise 2

 Online Activity—Preparing the Patient and Performing Respiratory Testing

 30 minutes

- Sign in to Mountain View Clinic.
- From the patient list, select **John R. Simmons**.
- On the office map, click on **Exam Room**.
- Click on the **Exam Notes** file folder on the counter to read the documentation regarding Dr. Simmons' visit.

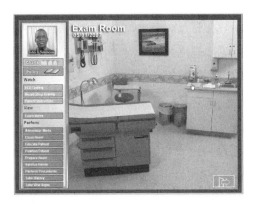

- Click **Finish** to close the Exam Notes and return to the Exam Room.
- Under the Watch heading, click on **Respiratory Testing** and watch the video.

1. What preparation of the patient was provided during the video?

 2. During the video, Dr. Simmons asked the medical assistant what the "contraption" was. At the time he asked this, what procedure was being performed—spirometry testing or peak flow monitoring? (*Hint:* Refer to Figure 27-15 and Figure 27-18 in your textbook to see illustrations of the devices used for each of these procedures.)

3. What were the physician's orders in regard to respiratory testing?

- Click the **X** in the upper right corner to close the video and return to the Exam Room.
- Click the exit arrow in the lower right corner of the screen to exit the room.
- On the Summary Menu, click **Return to Map** and select **Yes** at the pop-up menu to return to the office map.
- On the office map, click on **Billing and Coding**.
- Click on the **Encounter Form** clipboard on the counter to review the charges for peak flow monitoring or spirometry testing during Dr. Simmons' visit.

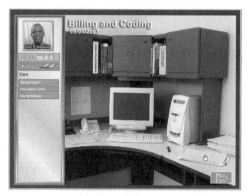

- Click **Finish** to close the Encounter Form and return to the Billing and Coding area.
- Click on **Charts** to open Dr. Simmons' medical record.
- Click on the **Patient Medical Information** tab and select **1-Progress Notes** from the drop-down menu.

4. For what procedure was Dr. Simmons charged? Is a specific place provided for peak flow monitoring on the Encounter Form?

Critical Thinking Question

5. Since spirometry testing and peak flow monitoring are both types of respiratory testing, could the physician have been more specific when writing the order? Should the Encounter Form be more specific by having respiratory testing as a heading that includes both peak flow monitoring and spirometry testing?

Critical Thinking Question

6. Assume that you are the Mountain View Clinic medical assistant responsible for reading the physician's order and the charges for Dr. Simmons' respiratory testing. Considering your review of the order and charges in the Encounter Form and Progress Notes, would you need to clarify what specific test the physician wanted performed? Explain your answer.

7. What is the proper position for spirometry testing? Why is the position important?

8. How many attempts should the patient be given to obtain quality spirometry testing?

9. During the testing, what should the medical assistant do to encourage an acceptable test?

10. Indicate whether each of the following statements is true or false.

   a. _____ During the video, the medical assistant provided the needed information for Dr. Simmons to obtain an acceptable test.

   b. _____ The patient's lips may be loosely pursed around the mouthpiece without affecting the results of the test.

   c. _____ To make the correct calculations when using a computerized spirometer, the medical assistant should obtain the patient's height and weight before performing the spirometry test.

   d. _____ When the test is completed, the mouthpiece may be reused.

   e. _____ The medical assistant should provide coaching only while the patient is exhaling air into the mouthpiece.

11. On the blank Progress Notes form below, document Dr. Simmons' respiratory testing, including his results of 250, 290, and 330.

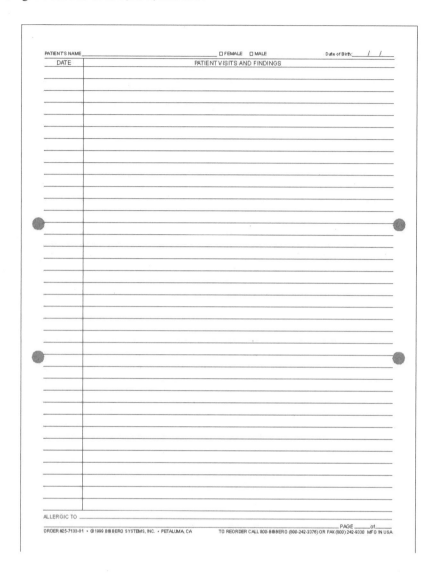

12. Continue reviewing the Mountain View Clinic medical assistant's written documentation of Dr. Simmons' testing in the Progress Notes. Compare this with your work in question 11. Which documentation do you think would be more helpful to the physician—the results as you documented them or the documentation by the Mountain View Clinic medical assistant in the Progress Notes?

 • Click **Close Chart** when finished to return to the Billing and Coding area.
   • Click the exit arrow in the lower right corner of the screen to exit the room.
   • On the Summary Menu, click **Return to Map** and select **Yes** at the pop-up menu to return to the office map.

Exercise 3

 Writing Activity—Peak Flow Measurement and Oxygen Therapy

10 minutes

1. Define *asthma*.

2. List some of the symptoms that a person with asthma experiences.

3. Identify some of the things that may trigger an asthma attack.

Critical Thinking Question

4. Ethan Griffin is a young patient at your clinic. He has chronic asthma and takes several medications to help control his asthma attacks. The physician has recommended that Ethan's parents use a peak flow meter at home. How would you explain to Ethan's parents the importance of performing the peak flow meter measurement and documenting his results for the medical office?

5. Give examples of when a patient might need home oxygen therapy.

Critical Thinking Question

6. After home oxygen therapy is initiated, how will the physician know whether the patient is responding?

7. What safety guidelines should be followed when a patient is prescribed home oxygen therapy?

19 ———————————————————

Fecal Specimen Collection

———————————————————————————————————————

Reading Assignment: Chapter 28—Specialty Examination and Procedures:
Colon Procedures, Male Reproductive Health, and
Radiology and Diagnostic Imaging

Patient: John R. Simmons

Learning Objectives:

- Understand the reasons for collecting fecal specimens.
- Use the package insert of a fecal occult test, and identify the correct steps to give to the patient when providing patient education for preparing and collecting the specimen.
- Describe the development of the fecal occult test and the visual appearance of the controls.
- Identify the possible indications of a positive fecal occult test.
- Understand the need for quality control when obtaining and testing a fecal specimen.

Overview:

In this lesson Dr. John R. Simmons, a college professor, will be asked to provide the medical office with fecal specimens to be tested for occult blood. The medical assistant has the responsibility of providing Dr. Simmons with the necessary information to ensure that a quality test will be obtained. Dr. Simmons has not been previously asked to collect for this test; consequently, specific instructions must be provided. Discussing fecal specimens tends to embarrass most patients, so it is important that the medical assistant respond with dignity and professionalism. When providing these instructions, giving correct instructions is imperative; otherwise, the patient may provide a specimen that cannot be tested.

Exercise 1

Online Activity—Patient Instruction for Collecting Fecal Specimens

 1 hour

- Sign in to Mountain View Clinic.
- From the patient list, select **John R. Simmons**.
- On the office map, click on **Exam Room**.
- Under the Watch heading, click on **Patient Instruction** and watch the video.

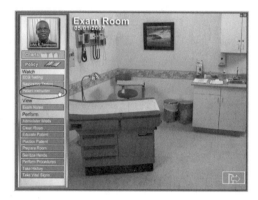

1. What is the primary purpose of a guaiac slide tests, and what specimen is used for this test?

2. What other conditions may cause blood in the stool and a positive result?

3. Explain the difference between occult blood and visible blood in a stool specimen.

4. Dr. Simmons seems embarrassed by the need to collect stool specimens. How did the medical assistant attempt to put him at ease?

→ • Click the **X** in the upper right corner to close the video and return to the Exam Room.
- Click the exit arrow in the lower right corner of the screen to exit the room.
- On the Summary Menu, click **Return to Map** and select **Yes** at the pop-up menu to return to the office map.

5. Which of the following supplies do patients need to obtain fecal specimens at home? Select all that apply. (*Hint:* Refer to Procedure 13-1 in your textbook if you need assistance.)

_____ Gloves

_____ Wooden applicator sticks

_____ Test kits (the number is based on the physician's policy)

_____ Plastic wrap

_____ Written instructions

_____ Envelope into which the cards are placed

Refer to the document "Stool Sample Insert" located in the Simulations folder on the Evolve site. Use this packet insert to answer the following questions. (*Note:* The kit described in this insert is just one type of fecal occult testing kit. You may need to use another type of kit with different directions where you work.)

6. Which of the following should the medical assistant tell the patient when providing instructions for preparing to obtain a fecal specimen? Select all that apply.

_____ Avoid all vegetables for 3 days.

_____ Eat a high-fiber diet for 3 days.

_____ Do not eat red meat, including processed meats and cold cuts, for 3 days.

_____ Take all medications ordered by the physician.

_____ Avoid taking aspirin, corticosteroids, and nonsteroidal antiinflammatory drugs (NSAIDs) for 1 week before collecting the specimen.

_____ Do not collect stool specimens during a menstrual period or for 3 days afterward.

_____ Eat foods that will cause a softening of stools to make the specimen easier to obtain.

_____ Eat small amounts of food that contain vitamin C.

_____ Do not eat raw fruits and vegetables, especially melons, radishes, turnips, and horseradish.

_____ Eat cooked vegetables.

_____ Drink at least three glasses of milk per day.

_____ Do not take iron or vitamin C for 3 days.

_____ Eat moderate amounts of bran cereal, popcorn, and other roughage.

7. When test kits are taken home, how should the patient store the kits until specimens are collected?

8. What directions should be given to the patient about the timing of specimens?

9. Which of the following are correct instructions to give to the patient about obtaining the stool specimen? Select all that apply.

_____ Using the wooden applicator stick, collect a sample of stool either from a container or from toilet paper.

_____ If the stool falls in the commode, collect the sample as you would from the container or the toilet paper.

_____ Open the flap of the first kit on the left (confirm that two square boxes are inside, labeled A and B); then smear a small amount of stool on the filter paper labeled A, making sure to spread it until thin.

_____ Using the same wooden stick, collect a second sample of stool from another area of the stool.

_____ Place this sample on top of the sample already collected.

_____ Place the second sample in the filter paper box labeled B.

_____ Close the front flap.

_____ Tear this test kit from the other two and place in the envelope provided.

_____ Add the date and time of collection on the flap.

_____ Repeat the same procedure with the next two stools (if three test kits are provided).

_____ Allow the specimens to air-dry before mailing them to the office.

_____ Place the specimens in a standard letter-sized envelope and mail.

_____ Place the specimens in an aluminum-lined envelope designed for sending these specimens to the medical office.

10. Why is it important to take the smears from two different areas of the stool?

11. Why is adding roughage to the patient's diet important?

12. On the following form, document the procedure for instructing the patient in the collection of a fecal specimen.

PATIENT'S NAME	☐ FEMALE ☐ MALE	Date of Birth: / /
DATE	PATIENT VISITS AND FINDINGS	

ALLERGIC TO

PAGE _____ of _____

ORDER #25-7133-01 • ©1999 BIBBERO SYSTEMS, INC. • PETALUMA, CA   TO REORDER CALL 800-BIBBERO (800-242-2376) OR FAX (800) 242-9330 MFG IN USA

Exercise 2

Writing Activity—Developing a Hemoccult Slide Test

30 minutes

A week after his visit, Dr. John R. Simmons has returned the Hemoccult slides to the medical office for development. In this exercise, you will describe the steps necessary to develop the test and provide documentation to the physician.

1. Which of the following supplies are needed for developing the Hemoccult test? Select all that apply.

   _____ Sterile gloves

   _____ Gloves

   _____ Gown and goggles

   _____ Developer solution

   _____ Wooden sticks

   _____ Watch

   _____ Reference card

   _____ Biohazard waste container

2. Now that you have chosen the proper supplies for developing the Hemoccult test, match the following columns to show the correct order of steps for the test.

Order	**Action**
_____ Step 1	a. Ensure quality control by checking the expiration date on slides and developer
_____ Step 2	
_____ Step 3	b. Don the correct personal protective equipment
_____ Step 4	c. Dispose of the used Hemoccult slides in the proper waste container
_____ Step 5	d. Read the results in 60 seconds
_____ Step 6	e. Open the back flap of slides
_____ Step 7	f. Document the results in the medical record
_____ Step 8	g. Sanitize hands after procedure
_____ Step 9	h. Sanitize hands before procedure
_____ Step 10	i. Compare the results with the reference card
	j. Apply two drops of developing solution to the guaiac test paper and the quality-control area

3. Why is reading the Hemoccult slide results at the end of 60 seconds important?

4. What is the volume of fecal blood loss that will result in a positive reading on the Hemoccult test?

5. The result of the first specimen obtained by Dr. Simmons was negative, but slides 2 and 3 were positive. Document these results on the following Progress Notes form.

| PATIENT'S NAME | ☐ FEMALE ☐ MALE | Date of Birth: / / |
| DATE | PATIENT VISITS AND FINDINGS | |

ALLERGIC TO _____

PAGE _____ of _____

ORDER #25-7133-01 • ©1999 BIBBERO SYSTEMS, INC. • PETALUMA, CA   TO REORDER CALL 800-BIBBERO (800-242-2376) OR FAX (800) 242-9330 MFG IN USA

6. What does a positive Hemoccult test indicate?

7. What are the indications if the positive quality-control area does not change to a blue color?

8. What are two possible causes of invalid tests?

9. What are possible causes of false-positive tests? (Hint: Refer to the package insert.)

10. Name two other types of stool tests that screen for colorectal cancer.

11. What are two differences between the fecal immunochemical test (FIT) and the guaiac slide test?

12. Have the advantages and disadvantages of the fecal DNA test been identified up to this point?

13. How does the fecal DNA test work?

14. Would the fecal DNA test be more expensive than the guaiac test?

Clean-Catch Urine

✐ **Reading Assignment:** Chapter 30—Urinalysis
- Collection of Urine
- Analysis of Urine

Patient: Louise Parlet

Learning Objectives:

- Discuss the reason for giving appropriate instructions to the patient before obtaining clean-catch midstream urine specimens.
- Identify the correct order of the steps needed to prepare either a male or a female patient for obtaining a clean-catch midstream urine specimen.
- Discuss how breaks in proper technique can lead to possible errors in diagnoses.
- Distinguish between correct and incorrect instructions for collecting a urine specimen.
- Complete a laboratory requisition form for a urine specimen.
- Understand the time limit for allowing urine to sit at room temperature before specimen integrity is compromised.

Overview:

Clean-catch midstream urine specimens are routinely obtained from patients for analysis for chemicals and possible bacteria. Since urinary catheterization is an invasive procedure, contamination by bacteria can be a problem. The clean-catch midstream procedure is the most effective means of obtaining a specimen that is as free of bacteria as possible. However, for the specimen to be of acceptable quality for examination, the patient must be given clear and specific instructions for collection. This lesson focuses on the medical assistant's role in providing patient education and ensuring the necessary steps for quality collection of a clean-catch midstream urine sample.

Exercise 1

Online Activity—Patient Education for Clean-Catch Midstream Urine Collection

 30 minutes

1. Why is providing proper patient education about the correct collection method for obtaining a clean-catch midstream urine specimen so important?

2. Indicate whether each one of the following statements is true or false.

   a. _____ All urine specimens collected in the medical office must be clean-catch midstream samples.

   b. _____ The container used to obtain a clean-catch midstream urine sample must be aseptically clean.

   c. _____ The clean-catch midstream procedure requires the patient to follow specific instructions when obtaining the specimen.

   d. _____ A clean-catch midstream urine sample is used to check for urinary tract infections.

   e. _____ The patient has the responsibility for the proper collection of the specimen.

   f. _____ Before collecting the specimen, a female patient should cleanse the perineum (pubis to anus) from back to front.

   g. _____ Before collecting the specimen, a male patient should cleanse by wiping down each side of the urinary meatus and then wiping directly across the urethral opening.

 • Sign in to Mountain View Clinic.
   • From the patient list, select **Louise Parlet**.
   • On the office map, click on **Exam Room**.
   • Under the Watch heading, click on **Urine Specimen Collection** and watch the video.

3. In the video, what incorrect information did the medical assistant given to the patient? What is the correct instruction?

• Click on the **Supply Cabinet**.

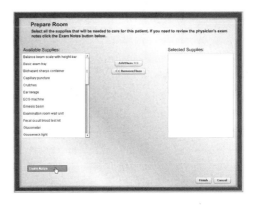

- Add the supplies needed for Louise Parlet's examination by clicking on the supply from the Available Supplies list and clicking **Add Item** to confirm your choice. The items you select will appear in the Selected Supplies box. When you click on an item, a photograph of that item will appear, which can be used for reference as you review your list of supplies. (*Note:* You can reopen the Exam Notes located in the lower left corner for reference as you make your selections.)

- If you wish to remove a chosen supply, highlight the item in the Selected Supplies box and click **Remove**.

- Repeat these steps until you are satisfied that you have everything you need from the list.

- Once you have made your selections, click **Finish** to return to the Exam Room.

- Click the exit arrow in the lower right corner of the screen to exit the room.

- On the Summary Menu, click on **Look at Your Performance** Summary.

- Scroll down the Performance Summary to the Prepare Room section and compare your answers with those chosen by the experts.

- You may save and print the Performance Summary for your records or turn it in to your instructor. The icons for saving and printing the Performance Summary are located at the top right corner of the screen.

- Click **Close** to return to the Summary Menu.

- On the Summary Menu, click **Return to Map** and select **Yes** at the pop-up menu to return to the office map.

4. Match the following columns to show the correct order of steps in the collection of a clean-catch midstream urine specimen for the female patient.

Order	Action
_____ Step 1	a. Pull undergarments down and sit on the toilet. Expose the urinary meatus by spreading apart the labia with one hand.
_____ Step 2	
_____ Step 3	b. Wash your hands and open the towelette packages and place them on the wrapper.
_____ Step 4	c. Cleanse each side of the urinary meatus with a front-to-back motion from pubis to the anus using a separate antiseptic wipe to clean each side of the meatus. After use, discard each towelette in the toilet.
_____ Step 5	
_____ Step 6	
_____ Step 7	d. Complete voiding (not into the container) into the toilet.
_____ Step 8	e. Void a small amount of urine, not catching the urine in the container.
_____ Step 9	f. Void into the container, collecting approximately one half of a cup of urine.
_____ Step 10	
_____ Step 11	g. Hold the container without touching the rim.
_____ Step 12	h. Wash your hands and return the specimen.
_____ Step 13	i. Open the collection container without touching the rim or inside of the cup or lid.

j. Close the container, taking care to not touch the rim or inside.

k. Cleanse down the center of the meatus from the front to the back.

l. Wash your hands.

5. Why should the patient be reminded to wash his or her hands before obtaining the specimen?

Critical Thinking Question

6. How can improper cleansing affect the integrity of the urine specimen? What implication can improper cleansing lead to in the treatment of the patient?

7. After the specimen has been collected, how long should it be allowed to stand before testing?

8. Why should the specimen be processed as quickly as possible?

Critical Thinking Question

9. The physician asks you to have Joe Smith collect a clean-catch midstream urine specimen before he leaves the office after an 11:30 appointment. You instruct Joe to bring the urine specimen into the laboratory when he has finished collecting the specimen. After you get back from lunch, you check the examination rooms and the patient restroom and find a container with urine in it sitting on the shelf in the bathroom. The cup is labeled Joe Smith. It is now 1:00 in the afternoon. What should you do?

10. What data should be included in charting the collection a clean-catch midstream urine specimen? Select all that apply.

_____ Date of collection

_____ Time of collection

_____ Time that the specimen was provided to the laboratory

_____ Type of specimen collected

_____ Instructions provided to the patient

_____ Type of test ordered

_____ Signature of person responsible for giving the patient instructions and processing the specimen

- On the office map, click on **Laboratory**.
- Click on **Collect Specimens** to collect the specimens that need to be tested for Louise Parlet.

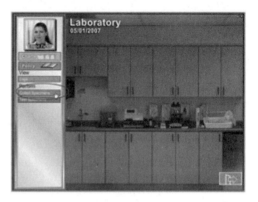

- Use the checkboxes to select the tests that need to be collected for Ms. Parlet's visit. (*Hint:* If you wish to review the notes for this visit, click on **Charts** on the Room Menu; then click on the **Patient Medical Information** tab and select **3-Progress Notes** from the drop-down menu.)
- Click **Next**.
- A series of questions will be asked for each test you selected. Use the checkboxes and radio buttons to answer all the questions related to each test you selected. (*Hint:* The Policy Manual can be opened at any time for reference as you answer the questions.)
- Click **Finish** to return to the Laboratory.
- Click on **Charts** to open the patient's medical record.
- Click on the **Patient Medical Information** tab and select **3-Progress Notes** from the drop-down menu.

11. Complete the following laboratory requisition form as ordered in the Progress Notes by Dr. Hayler.

Lab Services

IMPORTANT
Patient instructions and map on back

PHYSICIAN ORDERS

M ☐ Patient
F ☐ SS# ___ – ___ – ___

Patient _____ _____ _____   D.O.B. _____
        Last Name   First   M.I.

Address _____ City _____ Zip _____ Phone # _____

Physician _____
ATTACH COPY OF INSURANCE CARD

Date & Time of Collection:
_____
_____
Drawing Facility: _____

Diagnosis/ICD-9 Code _____
(Additional codes on reverse)

☐ ROUTINE   ☐ PHONE RESULTS TO: # _____
☐ ASAP   ☐ FAX RESULTS TO: # _____
☐ STAT   ☐ COPY TO: _____

☐ 789.00 Abdominal Pain
☐ 285.9 Anemia (NOS)
☐ 414.9 Coronary Artery Disease (CAD)
☐ 250.0 DM (diabetes mellitus)
☐ 780.7 Fatigue/Malaise
☐ 272.0 Hypercholesterolemia
☐ 244.9 Hypothyroidism
☐ 272.4 Hyperlipidemia
☐ 401.9 Hypertension
☐ 485.9 URI (upper respiratory infection)

HEMATOLOGY
☐ 1021 CBC, Automated Diff (incl. Platelet Ct.)
☐ 1023 Hemoglobin/Hematocrit
☐ 1020 Hemogram
☐ 1025 Platelet Count
☐ 1150 Pro Time Diagnostic
☐ 1151 Pro Time, Therapeutic
☐ 1155 PTT
☐ 1315 Reticulocyte Count
☐ 1310 Sed Rate/Westergren

URINE
☐ 1059 Urinalysis
☐ 1082 Urinalysis w/Culture if indicated
    Urine-24 Hr _____ Spot _____
    Ht. _____ Wt. _____
☐ 3033 Creatinine
☐ 3036 Creatinine Clearance (also requires blood)
☐ 3398 Protein
☐ 3096 Sodium/Potassium
☐   Microalbumin 24 Hr _____ Spot ____

SEROLOGY
☐ 8020 ANA (Antinuclear Antibody)
☐ 8040 Mono Spot
☐ 3494 Rheumatoid Factor
☐ 8010 RPR
☐ 5365 Rubella

CHEMISTRY
☐ 5550 Alpha Fetoprotein, Prenatal
☐ 3000 Amylase
☐ 3153 B12/Folate
☐ 3156 Beta HCG, Quantitative
☐ 3321 Bilirubin, Total
☐ 3324 Bilirubin, Total/Direct
☐ 3009 BUN
☐ 3159 CEA
☐ 3348 Cholesterol
☐ 3030 Creatinine, Serum
☐ 3509 Digoxin (recommend 12 hrs., after dose)
☐ 3515 Dilantin
☐ 3168 Ferritin
☐ 3193 FSH
☐ 3066 ▼ Glucose, Fasting
☐ 3061 Glucose, 1° Post 50 g Glucola
☐ 3075 ▼ Glucose, 2° Post Glucola
☐ 3060 Glucose, 2° Post Prandial (meal)
☐ 3049 ▼ Glucose Tolerance Oral GTT
☐ 3047 ▼Glucose Tolerance Gestational GTT
☐ 3650 Hemoglobin, A1C

CHEMISTRY
☐ 5232 HBsAg
☐ 3175 HIV (Consent required)
☐ 3581 Iron & Iron Binding Capacity
☐ 3195 LH
☐ 3590 Magnesium
☐ 3527 Phenobarbital
☐ 3095 Potassium
☐ 3689 Pregnancy Test, Serum (HCG, qual)
☐ 3653 Pregnancy Test, Urine
☐ 3197 Prolactin
☐ 3199 PSA
☐ 3339 SGOT/AST
☐ 3342 SGPT/ALT
☐ 3093 Sodium/Potassium, Serum
☐ 3510 Tegretol
☐ 3551 Theophylline
☐ 3333 Uric Acid

MICROBIOLOGY
Source _____
☐ 7240 Culture, AFB
☐ 7200 Culture, Blood x _____
☐   Draw Interval _____
☐ 7280 Culture, Fungus
☐   Culture, Routine
☐ 7005 Culture, Stool
☐ 7010 Culture, Throat
☐ 7000 Culture, Urine
☐ 7300 Gram Stain
☐ 7355 Occult Blood x _____
☐ 7365 Ova & Parasites x _____
☐ 7400 Smear & Suspension
        (includes Gram Stain/Wet Mount)
☐ 7060 Rapid Strep A Screen (Negs confir by cult)
☐ 7065 Rapid Strep A Screen only
☐ 7030 Beta Strep Culture
☐ 5207 GC by DNA Probe
☐ 5130 Chlamydia by DNA Probe
☐ 5555 Chlamydia/GC by DNA Probe
☐ 7375 Wright Stain, Stool

Additional Tests _____

PANELS & PROFILES

☐ X **3309 CHEM 12**
Albumin, Alkaline Phosphatase, BUN, Calcium, Cholesterol, Glucose, LDH, Phosphorus, AST, Total Bilirubin, Total Protein, Uric Acid

☐ ▼ **3315 CHEM 20**
Chem 12, Electrolyte Panel, Creatinine, Iron, Gamma GT, ALT, Triglycerides

☐ ▼ **3357 CARDIAC RISK PANEL**
Cholesterol, HDL, LDL, Risk Factors, VLDL Triglycerides

☐ X **3042 CRITICAL CARE PANEL**
BUN, Chloride, CO2, Glucose, Potassium, Sodium

☐ **3046 ELECTROLYTE PANEL**
Chloride, CO2, Potassium, Sodium

☐ ▼ **3399 EXECUTIVE PANEL**
Chem 20, Iron, Cardiac Risk Panel, CBC, RPR, Thyroid Cascade

☐ **5242 HEPATITIS PANEL, ACUTE**
HAVIgMAb, HBsAg, HBsAb, HBcAb, HCVAb

☐ ▼ **3355 LIPID MONITORING PANEL**
Cholesterol, Triglycerides, HDL, LDL, VLDL, ALT, AST

☐ **3312 LIVER PANEL**
Alkaline Phospatase, AST, Total Bilirubin, Gamma GT, Total Protein, Albumin, ALT

☐ X **3083 METABOLIC STATUS PANEL**
BUN, Osmolality (calculated), Chloride, CO2 Creatinine, Glucose, Potassium, Sodium, BUN/Creatinine, Ratio, Anion Gap

☐ X **3376 PANEL B**
Chem 12, CBC, Electrolyte Panel

☐ ▼ **3382 PANEL D**
Chem 20, CBC, Thyroid Cascade

☐ X **3388 PANEL F**
Chem 12, CBC, Electrolyte Panel, Thyroid Cascade

☐ ▼ **3391 PANEL G**
Chem 20, Cardiac Risk Panel, CBC, Thyroid Cascade

☐ ▼ **3393 PANEL H**
Chem 20, CBC, Cardiac Risk Panel Rheumatoid Factor, Thyroid Cascade

☐ ▼ **3397 PANEL J**
Chem 20, Cardiac Risk Panel

☐ **5351 PRENATAL PANEL**
Antibody Screen ABO/Rh, CBC Rubella, HBsAg, RPR
☐ 1059 with Urinalysis, Routine
☐ 1082 with Urinalysis w/Culture if indicated

☐ X **3102 RENAL PANEL**
Metabolic Status Panel, Calcium, Phosphorus

☐ **3188 THYROID CASCADE**
TSH, Reflex Testing

▼ - patient **required** to fast for 12-14 hours

X - patient recommended to fast 12-14 hours

LAB USE ONLY		INIT _____
☐ SST	☐ PLASMA	
☐ PURPLE	☐ SERUM	
☐ YELLOW	☐ SWAB	
☐ BLUE	☐ SLIDES	
☐ GREEN	☐ DNA PROBE	
☐ GREY	☐ B. CULT BTLS	
☐ URINE		
☐ BLACK		
☐ OTHER: _____		
REC'V. SPECIMEN:	☐ FROZEN	
☐ AMBIENT	☐ ON ICE	

Special Instructions/Pertinent Clinical Information _____

Physician's Signature _____   Date _____

These orders may be FAXed to: 449-5288

LAB

7060-500 (7/96)

12. Note that an order for a urine culture can be marked in two different places on the Laboratory Requisition. What is the difference between the two locations?

 • Click **Close Chart** when finished to return to the Laboratory.

• Click the exit arrow in the lower right corner of the screen to exit the room.

• On the Summary Menu, click on **Look at Your Performance Summary**.

• Scroll down the Performance Summary to the appropriate section and compare your answers with those chosen by the experts.

• You may save and print the Performance Summary for your records or turn it in to your instructor. The icons for saving and printing the Performance Summary are located at the top right corner of the screen.

• Click Close to return to the Summary Menu.

• On the Summary Menu, click **Return to Map**, then click **Yes** at the pop-up menu to return to the office map or click Exit the Program.

Urinalysis

🤓 **Reading Assignment:** Chapter 30—Urinalysis
- Composition of Urine
- Collection of Urine
- Analysis of Urine

Patient: Janet Jones

Learning Objectives:

- Identify the organs and main function of the urinary system.
- Discuss the reasons for performing a urinalysis.
- Identify the routine methods for collecting urine specimens in the physician's office laboratory setting.
- Describe the differences in testing results that can be expected with random and clean-catch midstream specimens.
- Describe the procedure for performing a dipstick urine specimen.
- List the three components included in a urinalysis.
- Prepare a laboratory requisition for a dipstick urinalysis.
- Discuss the determinants in the physical examination of urine.
- Explain the differences between qualitative and quantitative testing of urine.
- Describe the steps in quality control with urine testing.
- Document the instructions that should be given to the patient who is collecting a 24-hour urine specimen.

Overview:

This lesson is designed to reinforce the proper procedures for obtaining a clean-catch midstream urine specimen and then physical and chemical urinalyses. Janet Jones has a history of kidney disease and will need a urinalysis to provide a differential diagnosis for her back pain. As the medical assistant, you will be expected to understand the necessary information to perform a urinalysis, ensuring quality control.

Exercise 1

Writing Activity—Urine Components and Collection

25 minutes

1. On the diagram below, label the organs of the urinary tract. Use a text or online resource to assist if needed.

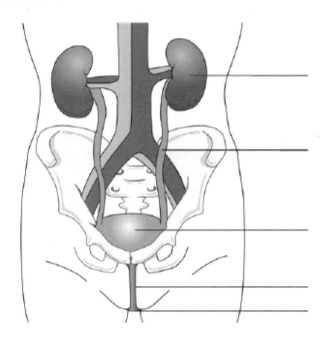

2. Which are valid reasons for performing urinalysis?
   a. For assessment of pathologic conditions in body systems
   b. As a screening measure for the possibility of pathologic conditions
   c. To assist in evaluation of the effectiveness of medical treatment
   d. For detection of abused substances
   e. All of the above

3. Match each of the following terms with its definition.

Term	Definition
_____ Hematuria	a. Secretion and passage of large amounts of urine
_____ Nocturia	b. Excessive urination of over 2000 mL in 24 hours
_____ Oliguria	c. Act of voiding urine
_____ Polyuria	d. Excessive urination during the night
_____ Micturition	e. Decreased output of urine volume
_____ Diuresis	f. Failure of the kidneys to produce urine
_____ Anuria	g. Blood present in urine

4. Which urine collection methods are routinely used for urinalysis in the medical office? Select all that apply.

_____ Random samples

_____ Last-voided specimen of the day

_____ 24-hour urine specimens

_____ Clean-catch midstream specimens

_____ Catheterized specimens

_____ Early-morning voided specimens

_____ First-voided morning specimens

_____ Sterile specimens

5. Which of the following are accurate, important guidelines when collecting a urine specimen? Select all that apply.

_____ Obtain a full cup of urine.

_____ Obtain 30 to 50 mL of urine.

_____ Label the specimen with only the patient's name.

_____ Label the specimen with the patient's name and the date and time of collection.

_____ Label the specimen with the patient's name, the patient's date of birth, the date and time of collection, and the type of specimen.

_____ Label the specimen with the patient's name, the date and time of collection, and the initials of the person handling the specimen.

_____ On the Laboratory Requisition form, record all medications the patient is taking.

_____ Avoid collecting urine from a patient during menstruation and a few days after menstruation, if possible.

_____ Allow time for the patient to void and supply water for the patient to drink if necessary.

_____ Do not allow the patient to leave the office until the specimen has been collected.

6. What instructions should be given to the patient for a 24-hour urine specimen?

Exercise 2

 Online Activity—Performing a Urinalysis

 25 minutes

1. What differences in test results could be expected with random-catch versus clean-catch midstream urine specimens?

- Sign in to Mountain View Clinic.
- From the patient list, select **Janet Jones**.
- On the office map, click on **Exam Room**.
- Under the Watch heading, click on **Specimen Collection** and watch the video.

Critical Thinking Question

2. After Ms. Jones listened to the directions for collecting a clean-catch midstream urine specimen, why do you think the medical assistant asked her to repeat the instructions just given to her?

• Click the **X** in the upper right corner to close the video and return to the Exam Room.
- Click the exit arrow in the lower right corner of the screen to exit the room.
- On the Summary Menu, click **Return to Map** and select **Yes** at the pop-up menu to return to the office map.
- From the office map, click on **Billing and Coding**.
- Click on **Charts** to open Janet Jones' medical record.
- Click on the **Workers' Comp** tab and select **2-Progress Notes** from the drop-down menu.

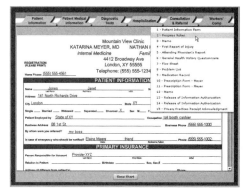

- Review the documentation in the Progress Notes regarding Ms. Jones' medical history.

3. Based on Ms. Jones' medical history, why would obtaining a urine specimen be important?

 • When finished, click **Close Chart** to return to the Billing and Coding area.

4. What is ureterolithiasis?

5. The three components of a urinalysis are _____, _____ , and _____ analysis of the urine.

6. In a urinalysis, what physical characteristics should be analyzed and documented?

7. Which of the following terms are acceptable to use for describing the appearance of urine? Select all that apply.

_____ Clear

_____ Smokey

_____ Bright

_____ Cloudy

_____ Hazy

_____ Misty

_____ Turbid (very cloudy)

_____ OK

8. Match each of the following abnormal colors of urine with its possible cause.

Abnormal Color	**Possible Cause**
_____ Orange	a. Fat droplets or pus
_____ Yellow-brown or green	b. Hemoglobin or red blood cells
_____ Red	c. Bile pigments
_____ Milky (white)	d. Pyridium

9. What are some of the causes of odoriferous urine?

10. Urine should have a slightly _____ odor.

11. Indicate whether each of the following statements is true or false.

a. _____ Cloudiness of urine is always a sign that the urine contains bacteria.

b. _____ Urine should be tested as soon as possible after collection.

c. _____ The smell of ammonia may be an indication of a urinary tract infection (UTI), because bacteria are breaking down urea in the specimen.

d. _____ The color of urine is caused by urochrome, which is produced from the breakdown of hemoglobin.

e. _____ The color of urine may vary from dark yellow to almost colorless.

f. _____ A milky appearance of urine may be caused by fat droplets or pus.

g. _____ Blood is always visually apparent in urine when present.

h. _____ Drugs do not have any effect on the color of urine.

i. _____ A musty smell to urine may come from foods eaten.

j. _____ A fruity odor to urine may be a sign of diabetes.

k. _____ The longer urine stands after collection, the more likely bacteria will grow.

l. _____ The specific gravity of urine measures the weight of urine compared with the weight of an equal volume of distilled water.

m. _____ Qualitative urine tests are useful for screening purposes, and quantitative test results indicate the exact amount of a chemical substance present in the body.

n. _____ Amphetamines, barbiturates, benzodiazepines, cocaine, marijuana, opiates, phencyclidine (PCP), methaqualone, and methadone are drugs (toxins) that can be identified by performing a rapid-drug screen.

12. Do you think that the medical assistant in the video was professional in providing information to Ms. Jones? Support your answer.

13. Other than the patient's medical history, what medical reason would Dr. Meyer have for obtaining a urine specimen from Ms. Jones?

14. When the chemical examination of urine is reported in amounts such as 1+, 2+, 3+, this is considered a _____ (**qualitative** or **quantitative**) testing of urine.

15. When the chemical examination of urine is reported in measurable units such as mg/dL, the test is reported as a _____ (**qualitative** or **quantitative**) test.

16. What procedure would you follow to perform the chemical analysis of Ms. Jones' urine specimen? (*Hint:* For this question, assume that you are opening a new bottle of reagent strips.)

17. Which of the following substances can be found on a dipstick urine reagent strip? Select all that apply.

    _____ Protein

    _____ Alcohol

    _____ Blood

    _____ White blood cells

    _____ Glucose or ketones

    _____ Urobilinogen

    _____ Bile

    _____ Bilirubin

    _____ Nitrite

    _____ pH (acidity or alkalinity)

    _____ Specific gravity

    _____ Color

18. Which of the following are proper guidelines for using reagent strips for urine testing? Select all that apply.

    _____ The specimen should be freshly voided.

    _____ Reagent strips may be used only with a clean-catch midstream specimen.

    _____ The specimen container should be clean.

    _____ The container should be free of detergent.

    _____ The container must be sterile.

_____ First-voided morning specimens may be desired for testing because they contain the greatest concentration of dissolved substances, and a small amount of an abnormal substance present in the specimen would be more easily detected.

_____ Specimens should be read against the color card for the test.

_____ When reading the test results, the amount of available lighting in the room is not important.

_____ Reagent strips may be stored under any conditions.

_____ The desiccant in the specimen bottle should remain in place until all strips have been used.

_____ It is best to store reagent strips in the refrigerator.

_____ Discoloration of the strips has no effect on testing.

_____ Quality control on the strips should be performed each day.

_____ Quality control ensures reliability of the test results.

19. Indicate whether each of the following statements concerning microscopic examination of specimens is true or false.

   a. _____ Microscopic examination of urine specimens is a Clinical Laboratories Improvement Act (CLIA)–waived test.

   b. _____ In urine, more than 5 red blood cells per high-power field is considered abnormal.

   c. _____ White blood cells are larger than red blood cells, are round and granular, and have a nucleus.

   d. _____ Squamous epithelial cells in urine are the result of sloughing of the outer layer of skin.

   e. _____ Squamous epithelial cells are not uncommon in urine specimens of women.

   f. _____ Renal epithelial cells are considered normal in a urine specimen.

   g. _____ Various crystals and casts may be found in urine.

   h. _____ Drugs (medications) may produce crystals in urine.

➤ • Click the exit arrow in the lower right corner of the screen to exit the Billing and Coding area.
   • On the Summary Menu, click **Return to Map** and select **Yes** at the pop-up menu to return to the office map.
   • On the office map, click on **Laboratory**.
   • Click on the **Specimen Collection Tray** to collect the specimens that need to be tested for Janet Jones.

- Use the checkboxes to select the tests that need to be performed with Ms. Jones' specimens. (*Hint:* If you wish to review the notes for this visit, click on **Charts** in the Room Menu, click on the **Workers' Comp** tab, and select **6-Progress Notes**.)
- Click **Next**.
- For each test you selected, a list of questions will appear. Answer all the questions related to each test, using the checkboxes and radio buttons provided. (Hint: The Policy Manual can be opened at any time for reference as you answer the questions.)
- Click **Finish** to return to the Laboratory.
- Next, click on the **Specimen Analyzer** to test Ms. Jones' specimens.

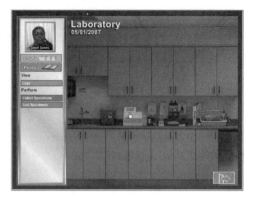

- Use the checkboxes to select the tests that need to be processed for Ms. Jones.
- Click **Next**.
- Questions will be asked for each test you selected. Answer all the questions related to each test, using the checkboxes and radio buttons provided. (*Hint:* The Policy Manual can be opened at any time for reference as you answer the questions.)
- Click **Finish** to return to the Laboratory.
- Click the exit arrow in the lower right corner of the screen to exit the Laboratory.
- On the Summary Menu, click on **Look at Your Performance Summary**.
- Scroll down the Performance Summary to the Collect Specimens section and the Test Specimens section and compare your answers with those chosen by the experts. Each test will have its own section.
- You may save and print the Performance Summary for your records or turn it in to your instructor. The icons for saving and printing the Performance Summary are located at the top right corner of the screen.

20. On the blank Progress Notes form below, document the following urine specimen testing results for Janet Jones (using today's date and time):

- The dipstick urine results are negative. The pH is 6.0, and the specific gravity is 1.020.
- Record the color as amber, and record the specimen as cloudy in appearance.

PATIENT'S NAME _____	☐ FEMALE ☐ MALE	Date of Birth: _/_/_
DATE	PATIENT VISITS AND FINDINGS	

ALLERGIC TO _____

PAGE ___ of ___

ORDER #25-7133-01 • ©1999 BIBBERO SYSTEMS, INC. • PETALUMA, CA   TO REORDER CALL 800-BIBBERO (800-242-2376) OR FAX (800) 242-9330 MFG IN USA

21. If Dr. Meyer had thought it necessary, she could have ordered a random urine specimen for Ms. Jones to be sent to the laboratory for a routine urinalysis with a microscopic and quantitative analysis. Prepare the following Laboratory Requisition form to order this test for the patient. Use today's date and the time of her appointment.

Lab Services

IMPORTANT
Patient instructions
and map on back

PHYSICIAN ORDERS

M ☐   Patient

Patient _____   _____   ___   D.O.B. _____   F ☐   SS# ___ – ___ – ___

           Last Name   First   M.I.

Address _____   City _____   Zip _____   Phone # _____

Physician _____

ATTACH COPY OF INSURANCE CARD

Date & Time of Collection:
_____ – _____

Drawing Facility: _____

Diagnosis/ICD-9 Code _____

(Additional codes on reverse)

☐ 789.00 Abdominal Pain   ☐ 414.9 Coronary Artery Disease (CAD)   ☐ 244.9 Hypothyroidism
☐ 285.9 Anemia (NOS)   ☐ 250.0 DM (diabetes mellitus)   ☐ 272.4 Hyperlipidemia
              ☐ 780.7 Fatigue/Malaise   ☐ 401.9 Hypertension
              ☐ 272.0 Hypercholesterolemia   ☐ 485.9 URI (upper respiratory infection)

☐ ROUTINE   ☐ PHONE RESULTS TO: # _____
☐ ASAP   ☐ FAX RESULTS TO: # _____
☐ STAT   ☐ COPY TO: _____

HEMATOLOGY	CHEMISTRY	CHEMISTRY	MICROBIOLOGY
☐ 1021 CBC, Automated Diff (incl. Platelet Ct.)	☐ 5550 Alpha Fetoprotein, Prenatal	☐ 5232 HBsAg	
☐ 1023 Hemoglobin/Hematocrit	☐ 3000 Amylase	☐ 3175 HIV (Consent required)	Source _____
☐ 1020 Hemogram	☐ 3153 B12/Folate	☐ 3581 Iron & Iron Binding Capacity	☐ 7240 Culture, AFB
☐ 1025 Platelet Count	☐ 3156 Beta HCG, Quantitative	☐ 3195 LH	☐ 7200 Culture, Blood x _____
☐ 1150 Pro Time Diagnostic	☐ 3321 Bilirubin, Total	☐ 3590 Magnesium	☐ Draw Interval _____
☐ 1151 Pro Time, Therapeutic	☐ 3324 Bilirubin, Total/Direct	☐ 3527 Phenobarbital	☐ 7280 Culture, Fungus
☐ 1155 PTT	☐ 3009 BUN	☐ 3095 Potassium	☐ Culture, Routine
☐ 1315 Reticulocyte Count	☐ 3159 CEA	☐ 3689 Pregnancy Test, Serum (HCG, qual)	☐ 7005 Culture, Stool
☐ 1310 Sed Rate/Westergren	☐ 3348 Cholesterol	☐ 3653 Pregnancy Test, Urine	☐ 7010 Culture, Throat
URINE	☐ 3030 Creatinine, Serum	☐ 3197 Prolactin	☐ 7000 Culture, Urine
☐ 1059 Urinalysis	☐ 3509 Digoxin (recommend 12 hrs., after dose)	☐ 3199 PSA	☐ 7300 Gram Stain
☐ 1082 Urinalysis w/Culture if indicated	☐ 3515 Dilantin	☐ 3339 SGOT/AST	☐ 7355 Occult Blood x _____
Urine-24 Hr _____ Spot _____	☐ 3168 Ferritin	☐ 3342 SGPT/ALT	☐ 7365 Ova & Parasites x _____
Ht. _____ Wt. _____	☐ 3193 FSH	☐ 3093 Sodium/Potassium, Serum	☐ 7400 Smear & Suspension
☐ 3033 Creatinine	☐ 3066 ▼ Glucose, Fasting	☐ 3510 Tegretol	(includes Gram Stain/Wet Mount)
☐ 3036 Creatinine Clearance (also requires blood)	☐ 3061 Glucose, 1° Post 50 g Glucola	☐ 3551 Theophylline	☐ 7060 Rapid Strep A Screen (Negs confir by cult)
☐ 3398 Protein	☐ 3075 ▼ Glucose, 2° Post Glucola	☐ 3333 Uric Acid	☐ 7065 Rapid Strep A Screen only
☐ 3096 Sodium/Potassium	☐ 3060 Glucose, 2° Post Prandial (meal)		☐ 7030 Beta Strep Culture
☐ Microalbumin 24 Hr _____ Spot _____	☐ 3049 ▼ Glucose Tolerance Oral GTT		☐ 5207 GC by DNA Probe
SEROLOGY	☐ 3047 ▼Glucose Tolerance Gestational GTT		☐ 5130 Chlamydia by DNA Probe
☐ 8020 ANA (Antinuclear Antibody)	☐ 3650 Hemoglobin, A1C		☐ 5555 Chlamydia/GC by DNA Probe
☐ 8040 Mono Spot			☐ 7375 Wright Stain, Stool
☐ 3494 Rheumatoid Factor			
☐ 8010 RPR			
☐ 5365 Rubella	Additional Tests _____		

PANELS & PROFILES

☐ ✗ **3309 CHEM 12**
Albumin, Alkaline Phosphatase, BUN, Calcium, Cholesterol, Glucose, LDH, Phosphorus, AST, Total Bilirubin, Total Protein, Uric Acid

☐ ▼ **3315 CHEM 20**
Chem 12, Electrolyte Panel, Creatinine, Iron, Gamma GT, ALT, Triglycerides

☐ ▼ **3357 CARDIAC RISK PANEL**
Cholesterol, HDL, LDL, Risk Factors, VLDL Triglycerides

☐ ✗ **3042 CRITICAL CARE PANEL**
BUN, Chloride, CO2, Glucose, Potassium, Sodium

☐ **3046 ELECTROLYTE PANEL**
Chloride, CO2, Potassium, Sodium

☐ ▼ **3399 EXECUTIVE PANEL**
Chem 20, Iron, Cardiac Risk Panel, CBC, RPR, Thyroid Cascade

☐ **5242 HEPATITIS PANEL, ACUTE**
HAVIgMAb, HBsAg, HBsAb, HBcAb, HCVAb

☐ ▼ **3355 LIPID MONITORING PANEL**
Cholesterol, Triglycerides, HDL, LDL, VLDL, ALT, AST

☐ **3312 LIVER PANEL**
Alkaline Phospatase, AST, Total Bilirubin, Gamma GT, Total Protein, Albumin, ALT

☐ ✗ **3083 METABOLIC STATUS PANEL**
Albumin, Osmolality (calculated), Chloride, CO2, Creatinine, Glucose, Potassium, Sodium, BUN/Creatinine, Ratio, Anion Gap

☐ ✗ **3376 PANEL B**
Chem 12, CBC, Electrolyte Panel

☐ ▼ **3382 PANEL D**
Chem 20, CBC, Thyroid Cascade

☐ ✗ **3388 PANEL F**
Chem 12, CBC, Electrolyte Panel, Thyroid Cascade

☐ ▼ **3391 PANEL G**
Chem 20, Cardiac Risk Panel, CBC, Thyroid Cascade

☐ ▼ **3393 PANEL H**
Chem 20, CBC, Cardiac Risk Panel, Rheumatoid Factor, Thyroid Cascade

☐ ▼ **3397 PANEL J**
Chem 20, Cardiac Risk Panel

☐ **5351 PRENATAL PANEL**
Antibody Screen ABO/Rh, CBC, Rubella, HBsAg, RPR
☐ 1059 with Urinalysis, Routine
☐ 1082 with Urinalysis w/Culture if Indicated

☐ ✗ **3102 RENAL PANEL**
Metabolic Status Panel, Calcium, Phosphorus

☐ **3188 THYROID CASCADE**
TSH, Reflex Testing

▼ - patient **required** to fast for 12-14 hours

✗ - patient recommended to fast 12-14 hours

LAB USE ONLY	INIT _____
☐ SST	☐ PLASMA
☐ PURPLE	☐ SERUM
☐ YELLOW	☐ SWAB
☐ BLUE	☐ SLIDES
☐ GREEN	☐ DNA PROBE
☐ GREY	☐ B. CULT BTLS
☐ URINE	
☐ BLACK	
☐ OTHER:	
REC'V. SPECIMEN:	☐ FROZEN
☐ AMBIENT	☐ ON ICE

Special Instructions/Pertinent Clinical Information _____

Physician's Signature _____   Date _____

These orders may be FAXed to: 449-5288

LAB

7060-500 (7/96)

Critical Thinking Question

22. If a patient is injured on the job, as Ms. Jones was, would you expect the employer to request a urine toxicology or drug screen on the employee after the injury occurred? Why or why not?

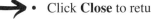

- Click **Close** to return to the Summary Menu.
- On the Summary Menu, click **Return to Map**, then click **Yes** at the pop-up menu to return to the office map or click **Exit the Program**.

Capillary and Venipuncture Procedures

👓 **Reading Assignment:** Chapter 24—The Pediatric Examination (Figure 24-16)
Chapter 29—Introduction to the Clinical Laboratory
Chapter 31—Phlebotomy

Patient: Kevin McKinzie

Learning Objectives:

- Identify the most commonly used venipuncture sites.
- Identify the types of specimens that can be obtained by venipuncture.
- Discuss the necessary preparation of the patient for a routine venipuncture.
- Determine what supplies are needed for a venipuncture.
- Review the need for standard precautions with venipuncture.
- Understand why proper positioning of the patient for venipuncture is necessary.
- Identify the process for safe capillary puncture on infants and older children or adults.
- Describe the equipment and supplies needed for capillary puncture.
- Identify the methods that can be used to increase blood flow when performing a capillary blood collection.
- Document the collection of the blood specimens.
- Indicate how to label and transport capillary specimens properly.

Overview:

This lesson reviews phlebotomy procedures, including venipuncture and capillary puncture, and discusses the importance of standard precautions and risk management skills to prevent injury to the patient. Using information obtained from the textbook, you will analyze proper techniques for venipuncture and capillary puncture, including proper positioning and educating the patient before the procedure and the proper selection of blood collection tubes for certain types of blood samples. After completing this lesson, you will have an understanding of the different types of blood specimens, as well as the proper disposal of contaminated supplies. Also discussed is proper site selection for capillary puncture and its importance in reducing patient discomfort and ensuring the safety of patients, especially infants.

Exercise 1

Online Activity—Identifying the Necessary Supplies for Venipuncture

20 minutes

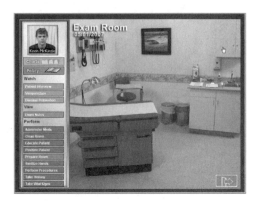

- Sign in to Mountain View Clinic.
- From the patient list, select **Kevin McKinzie**.
- On the office map, click on **Exam Room**.
- Click on the **Exam Notes** file folder to read the documentation regarding Kevin McKinzie's visit. Make note of any blood tests that will require phlebotomy during this visit.
- Click **Finish** to close the Exam Notes return to the Exam Room.
- Click on the **Supply Cabinet**.

- Add the supplies needed for Mr. McKinzie's examination by clicking on the supply from the Available Supplies list and clicking **Add Item** to confirm your choice. The items you select will appear in the Selected Supplies box. When you click on an item, a photograph of that item will appear, which can be used for reference as you review your list of supplies. (*Note:* You can reopen the Exam Notes located in the lower left corner for reference as you make your selections.)
- If you wish to remove a chosen supply, highlight the supply in the Selected Supplies box and click **Remove**.
- Repeat these steps until you are satisfied you have everything you need from the list.
- Once you have made your selections, click **Finish** to return to the Exam Room.
- Click the exit arrow in the lower right corner of the screen to exit the room.
- On the Summary Menu, click on **Look at Your Performance Summary**.
- Scroll down the Performance Summary to the Prepare Room section and compare your answers with those chosen by the experts.
- You may save and print the Performance Summary for your records or turn it in to your instructor. The icons for saving and printing the Performance Summary are located at the top right corner of the screen.
- Click **Close** to return to the Summary Menu.
- On the Summary Menu, click **Return to Map** and select **Yes** at the pop-up menu to return to the office map.

1. Which tests will require blood for completion of the physician's orders for the visit? Select all that apply.

_____ Urinalysis

_____ Complete blood count (CBC) with differential

_____ Hepatitis panel

_____ Liver panel

_____ Epstein-Barr virus (EBV) antibody

_____ MonoSpot test

2. Which of the tests you selected in question 1 would be sent to an outside lab for testing?

 Using your textbook for reference, decide what types of blood specimens will be needed for the ordered tests.

 • On the office map, click on **Laboratory**.
- Click on the **Specimen Collection Tray** to collect the specimens that need to be tested for Kevin McKinzie.
- Use the checkboxes to select the specimens that need to be collected for Mr. McKinzie's visit. (*Hint:* If you wish to review the notes for this visit, click on **Charts** in the Room Menu, click on the **Patient Medical Information** tab and select **1-Progress Notes**.)

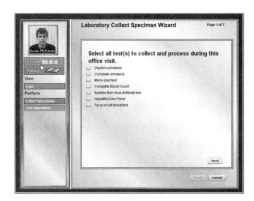

- Click **Next**.
- A series of questions will be asked for each test you selected. Answer all the questions related to each test, using the checkboxes and radio buttons provided. (*Hint:* The Policy Manual can be opened at any time for reference as you answer the questions.)
- Click **Finish** to return to the Laboratory.
- Click the exit arrow in the lower right corner of the screen to exit the room.
- On the Summary Menu, click on **Look at Your Performance Summary**.
- Scroll down the Performance Summary to the Laboratory Collection section and compare your answers with those chosen by the experts. Each test will have its own section.
- You may save and print the Performance Summary for your records or turn it in to your instructor. The icons for saving and printing the Performance Summary are located at the top right corner of the screen.

3. Indicate whether each one of the following statements is true or false.

a. _____ Serum is obtained from whole blood that has an anticoagulant added to the test tube to prevent clotting.

b. _____ Plasma is obtained from whole blood that has an anticoagulant added to the test tube to prevent clotting.

c. _____ Whole blood is needed for a CBC with differential.

d. _____ Serum is required for most blood chemistries and serology tests.

e. _____ A tube that has a clot activator would cause the patient's blood to clot faster than a tube without a clot activator.

f. _____ Inverting the tubes that have clot activators is not necessary to mix the clot activator with the blood specimen.

g. _____ Evacuated tubes are available in only one size.

h. _____ Evacuated tubes have an expiration date and a label for writing the patient's name.

i. _____ The needle within the Vacutainer should be pierced after the needle has entered the vein.

j. _____ If blood needs to be transferred from a syringe into a vacuum tube, then a needleless transfer device, such as a Hemoguard stopper, must be used, according to Occupational Safety and Health Administration (OSHA) requirements.

k. _____ Before using an evacuated tube, you should check it for cracks and other breaches in quality control.

l. _____ If a Vacutainer tube is dropped, it can still be used unless it is cracked or broken.

m. _____ The evacuated tube should be filled to the level of blood specified for the test, not to the size of the tube.

n. _____ Tubes containing additives should be agitated 8 to 10 times to mix the blood with the additive.

4. Tubes with or without a clot activator and tubes with or without a gel barrier are used to

   collect _____ specimens.

5. List the parts of the Vacutainer system.

6. Match the columns below to indicate the correct order of tubes to be used when drawing blood for testing.

Order	**Tube Stopper Color**
_____ First	a. Lavender top
_____ Second	b. Yellow top or sterile tube for blood cultures
_____ Third	c. Red top, red-gray top, or gold top for serum
_____ Fourth	d. Light green-gray, light green
_____ Fifth	e. Light blue top for coagulation studies
_____ Sixth	f. Green
_____ Seventh	g. Gray

Critical Thinking Question

7. If you were the medical assistant performing phlebotomy on Kevin McKinzie, which tube would be drawn first—the red-gray speckled stopper tube or the lavender stopper tube?

Critical Thinking Question

8. a. If the physician had also ordered a blood culture for Mr. McKinzie, which additional tube would be needed to be collected?

   b. Would this change the order of draw?

   c. Why or why not?

9. Explain the importance of following the correct order of draw to "preserve the specimen integrity."

10. Suppose you were a student at Mountain View Clinic and you were watching the medical assistant draw Mr. McKinzie's blood. You notice that the tubes are being drawn in an order that does not match the recommended order of draw (purple stopper first, then the yellow stopper, and then the gray-red stopper tube). What should you do?

• Click **Close** to return to the Summary Menu.
• On the Summary Menu, click **Return to Map**, then click **Yes** at the pop-up menu to return to the office map.

Exercise 2

 Online Activity—Choosing the Correct Position and Site for a Venipuncture

 15 minutes

1. As a medical assistant, you will decide on the proper site for venipuncture. On the following figures, label the venipuncture sites that are most appropriate for obtaining blood specimens.

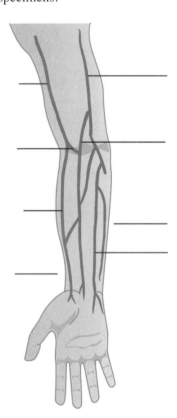
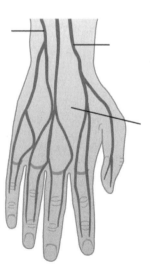

2. What are the advantages of using the veins found in the antecubital fossa?

3. If the veins are not easily palpable, what should be the next step in venipuncture?

→ • On the office map, click on **Exam Room**.
   • Under the Watch heading, click on **Venipuncture** and watch the video.
   • Click the **X** in the upper right corner to close the video and return to the Exam Room.

4. What additional steps should have been taken by the medical assistant to make the patient more at ease about the procedure?

5. Why is it important for the patient to be in either a lying or sitting position when being prepared for venipuncture?

6. What are other preparation steps for performing phlebotomy?

7. Indicate whether each one of the following statements is true or false.

a. _____   To successfully choose the best vein for performing phlebotomy, you must be able to see the vein (inspection).

b. _____   Sclerosed veins feel hard and knotty and should not be used for venipuncture.

c. _____   Veins that are near the top of the skin are always the best veins to use for venipuncture.

d. _____   The angle of the needle for venipuncture is 15 degrees.

e. _____   When blood is being drawn from the back of the hand, a butterfly needle or winged infusion set is more comfortable and more likely to provide a quality specimen.

f. _____   The tourniquet should be placed on the arm approximately 3 to 4 inches above the venipuncture site when finding the appropriate vein and should remain in place until after the venipuncture is complete, no matter how long the time.

g. _____   The tourniquet should remain in place until after the needle is removed after venipuncture.

→ • Remain in the laboratory with Kevin McKinzie and continue to the next exercise.

Exercise 3

Online Activity—Disposal of Supplies and Handling of Specimen Following Venipuncture

20 minutes

1. Name some of the supplies that are used during a phlebotomy.

2. After a venipuncture, what is the proper procedure for disposing the venipuncture supplies?

• Click on the **Waste Receptacles**.

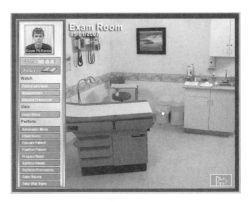

- Use the checkboxes to select the appropriate steps necessary to clean the Exam Room after Kevin McKinzie's examination.
- Click **Finish** to return to the Exam Room.
- Click the exit arrow in the lower right corner of the screen to exit the Exam Room.
- On the Summary Menu, click on **Look at Your Performance Summary**.
- Scroll down the Performance Summary to the Clean Room section and compare your answers with those chosen by the experts.
- You may save and print the Performance Summary for your records or turn it in to your instructor. The icons for saving and printing the Performance Summary are located at the top right corner of the screen.
- Click **Close** to return to the Summary Menu.
- On the Summary Menu, click **Return to Map** and select **Yes** at the pop-up menu to return to the office map.

3. Indicate whether each one of the following statements is true or false.

   a. _____ OSHA recommends that safety-engineered devices on needles be used to prevent needlestick injuries.

   b. _____ After venipuncture, all materials that have come in contact with the skin must be disposed of in the appropriate biohazard waste container.

   c. _____ OSHA requires that hands be sanitized after venipuncture.

   d. _____ The tourniquet used for the venipuncture should be sanitized using alcohol and then may be used for another patient, unless it is a disposable tourniquet, in which case it should be thrown away.

   e. _____ Gloves may be immediately removed after the venipuncture, and the test tubes with no gross contamination may be handled without gloves.

   f. _____ Handwashing or hand sanitization procedures should be performed after removing gloves and before documenting the procedure in the medical record.

   g. _____ The length of time a specimen is held after venipuncture and before centrifuging has no significant effect.

   h. _____ Specimens that are not handled with care may have hemolysis.

- On the office map, click on **Laboratory**.
- Click on **Charts** to open Kevin McKinzie's medical record.
- Click on the **Diagnostic Tests** tab and select **1-Laboratory Requisition** from the drop-down menu.
- Review the Laboratory Requisition to ensure that all tests that are not Clinical Laboratories Improvement Act (CLIA)-waived have been ordered.

4. Did you find that the tests were correctly ordered? Explain.

5. Should any of the tests have been collected on the *next* day because of the need to fast?

- When finished, click **Close Chart** to return to the Laboratory.
- Click on the **Lab Log Binder** to view the log of tests recently performed in the Laboratory.

6. Are all of the tests properly logged for quality control and for following the results of the tests?

7. Using the log below, document the specimens for Kevin McKinzie as found in the physician's notes. The requisition number is 144756.

Requisition Number	Date of Specimen Collection	Patient Name	Laboratory Test	Processing Lab	Initials: Specimen Collection	Date of Results Return	Initials: Results Return

- Click **Finish** to close the log and return to the Laboratory.
- Click on the **Specimen Analyzer** to test Kevin McKinzie's specimens.
- Use the checkboxes to select the tests that need to be processed for Kevin McKinzie.
- Click **Next**.

- A series of questions will be asked for each test you selected. Answer all the questions related to each test, using the checkboxes and radio buttons provided. (*Hint:* The Policy Manual can be opened at any time for reference as you answer the questions.)
- Click **Finish** to return to the Laboratory.
- Remain in the Laboratory with Kevin McKinzie and continue to the next exercise.

Exercise 4

Online Activity—Documentation of the Specimens

5 minutes

- Inside the laboratory, click on **Charts** to open Kevin McKinzie's medical record.
- Click on the **Patient Medical Information** tab and select **1-Progress Notes** from the drop-down menu to review information on where the specimen will be sent.

1. Mr. McKinzie's appointment time was 2:45 p.m. Using this information and the tests ordered, document on the following blank Progress Notes form the collection of the venipuncture specimens, including the laboratory to which the specimens were sent.

| PATIENT'S NAME | ☐ FEMALE ☐ MALE | Date of Birth: ___ / ___ / ___ |
| DATE | PATIENT VISITS AND FINDINGS | |

ALLERGIC TO _____

PAGE ____ of ____

ORDER #25-7133-01 • ©1999 BIBBERO SYSTEMS, INC. • PETALUMA, CA   TO REORDER CALL 800-BIBBERO (800-242-2376) OR FAX (800) 242-9330 MFG IN USA

2. What information is lacking from the documentation of the venipuncture in the medical record?

 3. What should be recorded on the tubes of blood before they are sent to the outside laboratory? (*Hint:* Refer to Figure 31-17 in the textbook if you need assistance.)

 • When finished, click **Close Chart** to return to the Laboratory.
• Click the exit arrow in the lower right corner of the screen to exit the Laboratory.
• On the Summary Menu, click **Return to Map**, then click **Yes** at the pop-up menu to return to the office map or click **Exit the Program**.

Exercise 5

 Writing Activity—Performing Capillary Puncture on Infants and Older Children or Adults

 15 minutes

 In this exercise, you will determine the proper site for capillary puncture for infants and other patients. (*Hint:* Refer to your textbook to complete the questions in this exercise.)

1. On the following figure, show the proper sites for adult capillary puncture.

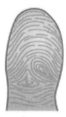

2. On the following figure, show the proper sites for infant capillary puncture.

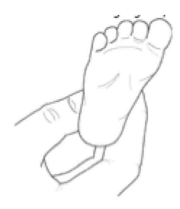

3. List situations when capillary puncture would be appropriate.

4. Indicate whether each one of the following statements is true or false.

a. _____ The site of puncture in an infant is an important factor in preventing the possibility of nerve damage.

b. _____ The site of puncture in an older child or an adult is an important factor in preventing the possibility of nerve damage.

c. _____ The proper selection of the puncture site for an adult prevents unnecessary discomfort.

d. _____ The length of the lancet to be used for adults and infants is the same.

e. _____ The same collection containers used for venipuncture may be used for capillary punctures.

f. _____ Capillary puncture is used to obtain small amounts of blood.

g. _____ Collection containers for capillary puncture have many of the same additives as those used for venipuncture.

h. _____ The plantar surface of the heel is used for puncture of infants who are not yet walking, but this is not the preferred site after the child begins walking.

i. _____ All fingers are acceptable sites for capillary puncture.

j. _____ Specimens obtained by capillary puncture should be handled as carefully as those from venipuncture to prevent hemolysis.

k. _____ Blood collected with a capillary puncture is pulled into the collection device either by capillary action or by being dropped onto a reagent strip for testing. It can also be collected with a microcollection device.

l. _____ Documentation of capillary puncture does not necessarily include the site of puncture, but this information should be included for infants.

m. _____ When specimens are collected by capillary puncture, the usual documentation needed for legal purposes is the type of test performed.

n. _____ The same safety precautions used with venipuncture should be used with capillary puncture.

o. _____ Because of the added chance of contamination of surfaces by blood, having extra supplies such as gloves, gauze pads, and disinfectant readily available is wise.

5. Capillary puncture is appropriate under which of the following conditions? Select all that apply. (*Hint:* Use your critical thinking skills when making your choices.)

_____ When only a small amount of blood is needed for the sample

_____ For the patient who is afraid of needles and prefers a capillary puncture to draw all specimens

_____ For older patients who have small rolling veins that are difficult to enter and for whom the test can be performed with a small amount of blood

_____ For pediatric patients who are not yet able to walk

_____ When frequent blood samples are needed, such as that needed for patients with diabetes

_____ For teenagers who simply prefer the capillary puncture for all testing

_____ For patients who are obese, who have scarring at the venipuncture sites, who have had mastectomies, or who are at risk for venous thrombosis

Critical Thinking Question

6. What do you think would be the most efficient way to transport a capillary tube or micro-collection container?

7. When you are collecting capillary blood, what would be one way to increase blood flow to the area?

LESSON 23

Hematology Testing

🕮 **Reading Assignment:** Chapter 29—Introduction to the Clinical Laboratory
- Laboratory Tests
- Types of Clinical Laboratories
- Clinical Laboratory Improvement Amendments
- Quality Control

Chapter 32—Hematology
- Components and Function of Blood
- Hemoglobin Determination
- Hematocrit
- White Blood Cell Count
- Red Blood Cell Count
- Red Blood Cell Indices
- White Blood Cell Differential Count

Patient: Louise Parlet

Learning Objectives:

- Understand the three levels of laboratory testing as defined by the Clinical Laboratories Improvement Act (CLIA).
- List methods for obtaining specimens for CLIA-waived hematology testing.
- Read Progress Notes correctly.
- List the normal reference ranges for components of blood that are tested in a complete blood count (CBC).
- Discuss the role of the hematology section of the laboratory.
- Describe the collection of blood in a hematocrit (Hct) tube.
- Explain what is indicated by *MCH*, *MCV*, and *MCHC*.
- Document laboratory test results on a laboratory flow sheet.

Overview:

This lesson focuses on the importance of understanding CLIA-waived tests and hematology testing. You will use the Policy Manual to obtain the list of diagnostic tests for a patient, Louise Parlet, with a newly diagnosed pregnancy. You will also be expected to add hematology test results to a flow sheet for this patient.

Exercise 1

 Online Activity—Performing Diagnostic Tests According to Office Policy

30 minutes

- Sign in to Mountain View Clinic.
- From the patient list, select **Louise Parlet**.
- On the office map, click on **Exam Room**.
- Click on the **Exam Notes** file folder to read the documentation regarding Louise Parlet's visit. Make a notation of her primary diagnosis and the reason she is being seen in the office.

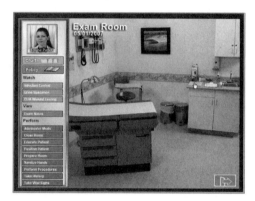

- Click **Finish** to close the Exam Notes and return to the Exam Room.
- Click on **Policy** to open the office Policy Manual.
- Select **Policy Manual**, "standing orders" in the search bar, and click on the magnifying glass.
- Read the section of the Policy Manual regarding standing orders.
- Keep the Policy Manual open to answer the following questions.

1. For what reason is Ms. Parlet being seen at the office today?

2. According to office Policy Manual, what measurements and tests should be obtained from Ms. Parlet?

→ • Click **Close Manual** to return to the Exam Room.

3. What is meant by *CLIA*?

4. What are the three levels of CLIA testing?
   a. Simple, moderate, and high complexity
   b. Waived, easy, and high complexity
   c. Waived, moderate, and high complexity
   d. Easy, medium, and complex complexity
   e. Waived, medium, and complex complexity

5. Indicate whether each of the following statements is true or false.

   a. _____ CLIA-waived tests include those tests that could be performed by the patient.

   b. _____ CLIA-waived tests are of moderate complexity.

   c. _____ The majority of medical offices perform waived tests.

   d. _____ CLIA-waived tests are approved by the United States Food and Drug Administration (FDA).

   e. _____ CLIA-waived tests are the most commonly performed laboratory tests in a hospital laboratory.

   f. _____ Many CLIA-waived test results can be determined by a color reaction.

   g. _____ Moderately complex CLIA testing must be performed by specially trained laboratory personnel.

   h. _____ Group A rapid streptococcus (strep) testing, dipstick urinalysis, urine pregnancy testing, and fecal occult blood tests are all CLIA-waived tests that can be performed in the medical office.

   i. _____ Microscopic analysis of urine is a CLIA-waived test.

   j. _____ A chemistry profile performed on a nonwaived automated blood analyzer would be included on the list of CLIA-waived tests.

   k. _____ CLIA testing requires quality control, quality assurance, and proficiency testing.

   l. _____ Quality control involves testing equipment for efficiency.

   m. _____ Quality assurance is the performance of tests to ensure the accuracy and reliability of the test results.

   n. _____ Proficiency testing is a form of external quality control designed to ensure that the equipment and supplies being used are reliable and meet nationally accepted standards.

6. List at least four methods for obtaining CLIA-waived tests.

7. Which of the tests identified in question 2 could be collected and performed by the medical assistant as CLIA-waived tests before the physician sees Ms. Parlet?

 • Click the **exit arrow** in the lower right corner of the screen to exit the Exam Room.
 • On the Summary Menu, click **Return to Map** and select **Yes** at the pop-up menu to return to the office map.
 • On the office map, click on **Billing and Coding**.
 • Click on **Charts** to open Louise Parlet's medical record.
 • Click on the **Patient Medical Information** tab and select **3-Progress Notes** from the drop-down menu.
 • Read the final Progress Notes for Ms. Parlet's visit.

8. According to the Progress Notes, what further blood tests were ordered for Ms. Parlet? Were any of these CLIA-waived tests?

9. Do the Progress Notes indicate that all the specimens were sent to QualityLab?

 • Click **Close Chart** when finished to return to the Billing and Coding area.
 • Click the exit arrow in the lower right corner of the screen to exit the room.
 • On the Summary Menu, click **Return to Map**, then click **Yes** at the pop-up menu to return to the office map or click **Exit the Program**.

Exercise 2

Writing Activity—Components of Hematology

30 minutes

In this exercise, you will review hematology, its components, and normal reference ranges for adult patients.

1. Define *hematology* and explain the responsibilities of the hematology section of the laboratory.

2. Match each of the following tests with its purpose (that is, the information it provides to the physician to help in diagnosing conditions and diseases).

Test		**Purpose**
_____ White blood cell (WBC) count		a. Measures (indirectly) the oxygen-carrying capacity of the blood
_____ Red blood cell (RBC) count		
_____ Platelet count		b. Measures the percentage of packed RBCs in a specimen
_____ Hct		c. Measures the number of erythrocytes in whole blood
_____ Hgb		d. Measures the approximate number of leukocytes in the circulating blood
		e. Measures the number of thrombocytes that aid in blood clotting

3. Define *MCV*, *MCH*, and *MCHC*. What is measured by each? (*Hint:* Use online resources if you need assistance.)

4. For each blood component listed below, identify the normal range for male and female patients.

Blood Component	Normal Range by Gender
RBCs (erythrocytes)	
WBCs (leukocytes)	
Hgb	
Hct	
WBC differential	

5. Describe the collection of a capillary puncture specimen in a calibrated capillary tube for a spun microhematocrit.

6. What should the medical assistant do if air bubbles are present in the capillary tube?

7. Why is it important for no air bubbles to be in the capillary puncture specimen for a spun Hct?

8. On the following diagram, label the cellular elements found in a capillary tube after centrifuging.

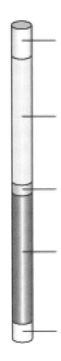

9. When a capillary tube is being spun in a microhematocrit centrifuge, which of the following steps are necessary for safety? Select all that apply.

_____ Wearing personal protective equipment (PPE)

_____ Placing a capillary tube anywhere in the centrifuge

_____ Placing capillary tubes opposite each other for balance

_____ Placing the sealed edge of the capillary tube toward the exterior of the centrifuge

_____ Placing the capillary tube toward the center of the centrifuge

_____ Closing the lid of the centrifuge before spinning the capillary tube

_____ Opening the lid immediately after the centrifuge stops the cycle

_____ Opening the lid when the centrifuge stops spinning

Exercise 3

Writing Activity—Documenting Hematology Testing

30 minutes

In this exercise, you will document Louise Parlet's laboratory results in her Progress Notes and on a flow sheet.

1. The only CLIA-waived test documented for Ms. Parlet was her urine hCG. Her Hgb, glucose level, and dipstick urine were also tested, but they were not documented until after the patient left the office at 9:45 am. On the blank Progress Notes below, document the following CLIA-waived test results for Ms. Parlet:

   - Hgb: 11.2 g/dL
   - Blood glucose: 115 mg/dL (nonfasting)
   - Dipstick urine: negative for glucose and albumin (protein) and leukocytes
   - pH: 7
   - Specific gravity: 1.025

PATIENT'S NAME	☐ FEMALE ☐ MALE	Date of Birth: __/__/__
DATE	PATIENT VISITS AND FINDINGS	

ALLERGIC TO _____

ORDER #25-7138-01 • ©1999 BIBBERO SYSTEMS, INC. • PETALUMA, CA   TO REORDER CALL 800-BIBBERO (800-242-2376) OR FAX (800) 242-9330. MFG IN USA   PAGE ____ of ____

2. Now fill in the results from the CLIA-waived testing performed during Ms. Parlet's visit on the following flow sheet.

FLOW SHEET

Name: *Louise Parlet* _____ Date of Birth: *07/04/1982* Age: *23*

Vital Signs	Date:	05/01/07								
Weight		125 lbs								
Height		5 ft 5 in								
Temperature		98.2 F								
Pulse		72								
Respirations		16								
Blood Pressure		104/72								
Lab Tests	**Date:**	05/01/07								
CBC										
RBC										
WBC										
HGB										
Hematocrit										
AlkalinePhosphatase										
Albumin										
Glucose										
Bilirubin total										
BUN										
Calcium										
Cholesterol										
Chloride										
CO2										
Creatinine										
Hb A1c										
LipidProfile										
LDL										
HDL										
Triglycerides										
SGGT										
SGOG/AST										
SGPT/ATL										
LDH										
T3										
T4										
T7										
TSH										
Triglycerides										
Total Protein										
Uric Acid										
Sodium										
Potassium										
Urinalysis										
Albumin										
Glucose										
PAPSmear										
PSA										
Other tests:										

3. Dr. Hayler received a partial report on Ms. Parlet's laboratory results today. Document the results in the following blank Progress Notes, using today's date and time and the following results:

- Hgb: 10.6
- Hct: 38%
- RBC count: 4.2:
- WBC count: 5400
- Platelet count: 200,000
- Pregnancy test: positive
- Rubella titer: 1:1 (assumed immune)
- ABO: O
- Rh: positive
- Papanicolaou (Pap) test: negative
- Chlamydia: negative

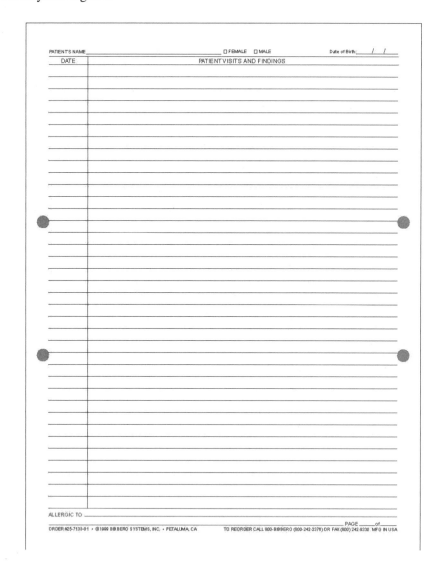

4. Begin documenting the laboratory results from the Progress Notes in question 3 onto the following flow sheet.

FLOW SHEET

Name: _Louise Parlet_   Date of Birth: _07/04/1982_ Age: _23_

Vital Signs	Date:	05/01/07										
Weight		125 lbs										
Height		5 ft 5 in										
Temperature		98.2 F										
Pulse		72										
Respirations		16										
Blood Pressure		104/72										
Lab Tests	Date:	05/01/07										
CBC												
RBC												
WBC												
HGB												
Hematocrit												
AlkalinePhosphatase												
Albumin												
Glucose												
Bilirubin total												
BUN												
Calcium												
Cholesterol												
Chloride												
CO2												
Creatinine												
Hb A1c												
LipidProfile												
LDL												
HDL												
Triglycerides												
SGGT												
SGOG/AST												
SGPT/ATL												
LDH												
T3												
T4												
T7												
TSH												
Triglycerides												
Total Protein												
Uric Acid												
Sodium												
Potassium												
Urinalysis												
Albumin												
Glucose												
PAPSmear												
PSA												
Other tests:												

5. Should any of Ms. Parlet's laboratory test results be highlighted for the physician for special attention? If so, which one(s)?

LESSON 24

Performing Blood Chemistry Testing

✏ Reading Assignment: Chapter 33—Blood Chemistry and Immunology

Patient: Rhea Davison

Learning Objectives:

- List the Clinical Laboratories Improvement Act (CLIA)-waived chemistry tests commonly performed in a medical office.
- Discuss the necessity of quality control for blood glucose tests in home and office testing.
- Identify the normal ranges of more commonly performed blood chemistry testing.
- Discuss the needed patient preparation for a fasting blood glucose and cholesterol test.
- Indicate which tests should be obtained as fasting blood chemistry tests when possible.
- State the patient teaching that is important when helping a patient to learn how to obtain blood glucose tests using a home glucose meter, such as Accu-Chek.
- List the supplies that are needed for blood glucose testing.
- Identify the side effects that may be experienced by patients when performing glucose tolerance tests.
- Describe the proper storage of blood glucose testing supplies.
- Complete the laboratory log for specimens being sent to an outside laboratory.
- Document the test results on a laboratory flow sheet and indicate those test results that need to be seen by the physician as soon as possible.

Overview:

In this lesson you will describe the collection and handling of some of the common CLIA-waived blood chemistry tests performed in the medical office. The normal range of blood chemistry results will be identified, and the ability to evaluate the test results will be emphasized. You will be expected to complete a laboratory log for specimens being sent to outside laboratories for testing. You will also document the return of the test results to the office. As the medical assistant, you will be asked to determine which results need immediate attention and which can be seen by the physician at the end of the day. Rhea Davison is an established patient with a known history of diabetes mellitus. She has kept her diabetes well controlled until her last visit. The physician is concerned that the glucose meter (glucometer) she is using at home may be providing inaccurate results, so you are asked to assist Ms. Davison in learning how to perform routine maintenance on the glucose meter.

Exercise 1

Writing Activity—Common Blood Chemistry Testing

20 minutes

1. What is measured through blood chemistry testing?

2. What is the most common type of specimen collected for a blood chemistry test that is performed at an outside laboratory?

3. Identify the CLIA-waived blood chemistry tests that are commonly performed in the medical office laboratory.

4. What patient preparation is needed for blood cholesterol and fasting glucose chemistry testing in the medical office?

5. What is the best appointment time for the patient to have a blood chemistry test?

6. Give the normal ranges for the following blood chemistry components.

   Blood urea nitrogen (BUN):

   Fasting blood glucose:

   Two-hour postprandial blood sugar (PPBS):

   Total cholesterol:

   High-density lipoprotein (HDL) cholesterol:

   Triglycerides:

7. When a glucose tolerance test is performed, what is the patient given to drink after the fasting glucose level is drawn?

8. What are some normal side effects that may occur in a patient who is having a glucose-tolerance test?

9. What are some more serious symptoms that, if experienced by the patient, may need to be reported to the physician immediately?

10. Provide the blood glucose average (in mg/dL) that correlates with each of the following glycosylated hemoglobin results (hemoglobin A1c):

    12.0:

    11.0:

    10.0:

    9.0:

    8.0:

    7.0:

    6.0:

    5.0:

    4.0:

Exercise 2

Online Activity—Patient Education for Quality Blood Glucose Tests

30 minutes

- Sign in to Mountain View Clinic.
- From the patient list, select **Rhea Davison**.
- On the office map, click on **Exam Room**.
- Click on the **Exam Notes** file folder to read the initial documentation regarding Rhea Davison's visit.

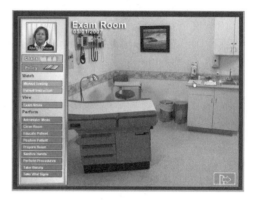

- Click **Finish** to close the Exam Notes and return to the Exam Room.
- Under the Watch heading, click on **Waived Testing** and watch the video.
- Click the **X** in the upper right corner to close the video and return to the Exam Room.

1. Now that you have read the Exam Notes and watched the video, why do you think that Dr. Meyer wants Ms. Davison to perform a glucose test using the equipment in the office?

 • Click on the **Supply Cabinet**.

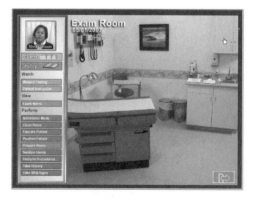

- Add the supplies needed for Rhea Davison's examination by clicking on the supply from the Available Supplies list and clicking **Add Item** to confirm your choice. The items you select will appear in the Selected Supplies box. When you click on an item, a photograph of that item will appear, which can be used for reference as you review your list of supplies. (*Note:* You can reopen the Exam Notes located in the lower left-hand corner for reference as you make your selections.)

• If you wish to remove a chosen supply, highlight the supply in the Selected Supplies box and click **Remove**.

• Repeat these steps until you are satisfied that you have everything you need from the list.

• Once you have made your selections, click **Finish** to return to the Exam Room.

2. List the supplies needed by a medical assistant for blood glucose testing.

3. Which of the following supplies would be needed by Ms. Davison to perform quality control of the glucose testing equipment she currently uses at home? Select all that apply.

_____ Abnormal control sample

_____ Gloves

_____ Normal control sample

_____ Glucose meter

_____ Sterile wipes

_____ Container for sharps

_____ Glucose reagent strips

_____ Capillary lancet

4. Indicate whether each of the following statements is true or false.

a. _____ All blood chemistry tests results are confined to only a single number for normal readings.

b. _____ Cholesterol and blood glucose may be CLIA-waived tests.

c. _____ To perform cholesterol and blood glucose testing in the medical office, the equipment must be CLIA-waived unless highly qualified personnel are available for the testing.

d. _____ At home, a patient should store equipment away from light and heat sources.

e. _____ Quality control is an important aspect of every laboratory test, including glucose testing.

f. _____ If a patient's hemoglobin A_{1c} level is high, the physician may need to change the patient's medication or investigate whether the patient is following instructions for managing his or her diabetes.

    g. _____ Blood chemistry testing is used for differential diagnoses.

    h. _____ The equipment used by patients at home is CLIA-waived.

    i. _____ All types of blood glucose equipment have the same instructions for use.

5. What information needs to be communicated to Ms. Davison about the collection of the specimen immediately after the capillary puncture?

6. What information should be communicated to Ms. Davison about the use of the glucose meter?

7. The medical assistant suggests that Ms. Davison ask the physician for a new glucose testing meter. Why do you think this request is important?

8. In the Exam Notes, Ms. Davison reports having missed several doses of medication because of an inability to buy the medication. How would you expect this fact to affect the test results she obtained at home?

9. Would you expect Ms. Davison to have an increase in weight if she is following her prescribed diet? Explain your answer.

10. What information did Ms. Davison give about where she stores her glucose meter? What affect may this fact have on the results of her tests?

- Click the exit arrow in the lower right corner of the screen to exit the Exam Room.
- On the Summary Menu, click on **Look at Your Performance Summary**.
- Scroll down the Performance Summary to the Prepare Room section and compare your answers with those chosen by the experts.
- You may save and print the Performance Summary for your records or turn it in to your instructor. The icons for saving and printing the Performance Summary are located at the top right corner of the screen.
- Click **Close** to return to the Summary Menu.
- On the Summary Menu, click **Return to Map** and select **Yes** at the pop-up menu to return to the office map.
- On the office map, click on **Check Out**.
- Click on **Charts** to open Rhea Davison's medical record.

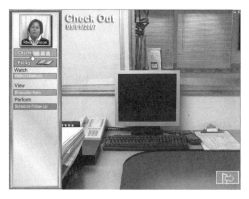

- Click on the **Patient Medical Information** tab and select **1-Progress Notes** from the drop-down menu.
- Read the results of today's blood glucose test and note the testing that is to be performed on the next day.
- Leave the patient's chart open as you answer the following questions.

11. Are the test results obtained in the office for Ms. Davison's blood glucose within the limits expected when compared with the results from her home testing? Explain your answer.

12. Dr. Meyer ordered a hemoglobin A_{1c} test. What information does this test provide? Why is this an important test for Dr. Meyer to use in treating Ms. Davison?

- Stay in the Check Out area with Rhea Davison as your patient. Leave the patient's chart open to use as a reference when you get to Exercises 4 and 5.

Exercise 3

Writing Activity—Quality Control with Blood Chemistry Testing

15 minutes

In this exercise you will use your knowledge to determine whether quality control has been accomplished.

1. Indicate whether each of the following statements is true or false.

   a. _____ Quality control for blood chemistry testing should be performed no more than once a day.

   b. _____ When new reagent strips are opened, quality control sampling should occur.

   c. _____ Quality control samples have expiration dates.

   d. _____ Quality control samples may be used with any equipment, regardless of the testing method.

   e. _____ Quality control is performed only to enable the physician to arrive at an accurate reading for comparison.

   f. _____ If the quality control samples are consistently inaccurate, the patient should try to repair the equipment used at home, because the patient is the person who best understands how that specific equipment works.

   g. _____ One method of checking for quality control of a machine in the medical office is to compare results obtained from a reference laboratory on a specific specimen with the results obtained on that same specimen in the office laboratory.

2. What is the significance if a sample used for quality control falls out of the control range?

Critical Thinking Question

3. If a patient complains about "the extra expense" of measuring his or her own blood glucose levels at home daily, what would be your response?

4. If a patient questions the need for performing quality control on a regular basis, what reasons could you provide to this patient?

Exercise 4

  Online Activity—Preparing a Laboratory Log for Patient Specimens

10 minutes

- Continue your care for Rhea Davison in the Check Out area at Mountain View Clinic. (*Note:* If you have exited the program, sign in again to Mountain View Clinic, select Rhea Davison, go to the Check Out area, and open the Progress Notes in her chart.)

1. Rhea Davison's specimens were sent to an outside laboratory (QualityLab) the day after her appointment. Using her Progress Notes, prepare the following laboratory log for these tests. The requisition number is 112417.

Requisition Number	Date of Specimen Collection	Patient Name	Laboratory Test	Processing Lab	Initials: Specimen Collection	Date of Results Return	Initials: Results Return
112417							

Exercise 5

 Online Activity—Adding Laboratory Results to the Flow Sheet

 20 minutes

- Continue documenting the results of Rhea Davison's blood chemistry test in the medical record. (*Note:* If you have exited the program, sign in again to Mountain View Clinic, select Rhea Davison, go to the Check Out area, and open the Progress Notes in her chart.)

1. Using the blank flow sheet on the next page, transfer the test results recorded in Ms. Davison's Progress Notes for 5/1/07. In addition, add the following results, which were received by Dr. Meyer on 5/3/07:

Blood Chemistry

- Alkaline phosphatase: 4
- Bilirubin: 1.2
- Serum glutamic oxaloacetic transaminase (SGOT): 14
- Bicarbonate (CO_2): 21
- Calcium: 7.2
- Chloride: 98
- Creatinine: 0.6
- Lactate dehydrogenase (LDH): 96
- Glucose: 460
- Potassium: 4.8
- Total protein: 6.6
- Sodium: 130
- BUN: 18
- Phosphorus: 3.2

Thyroid Profile

- Thyroxine (T_4): 10.8
- Triiodothyronine (T_3): 185
- Thyroid-stimulating hormone (TSH): 15.4 (normal values)
- Cancer antigen (CA) 125: 3.6 (abnormal value)
- Hemoglobin A_{1c}: 10 (abnormal value)

FLOW SHEET

Name: Rhea Davison   Date of Birth: 08/16/1953   Age: 53

Vital Signs Date:	05/01/07									
Weight	152									
Height	5 ft 1 in									
Temperature	98.6									
Pulse	86									
Respirations	24									
Blood Pressure	144/86									
Lab Tests Date:										
CBC										
RBC										
WBC										
HGB										
Hematocrit										
Alkaline Phosphatase										
Albumin										
Glucose										
Bilirubin total										
BUN										
Calcium										
Cholesterol										
Chloride										
CO2										
Creatinine										
HgbA1c										
Lipid Profile										
LDL										
HDL										
Triglycerides										
SGOT										
SGOG/AST										
SGPT/ATL										
LDH										
T3										
T4										
T7										
TSH										
Triglycerides										
Total Protein										
Urea Nitrogen										
Sodium										
Potassium										
Urinalysis										
Albumin										
Glucose										
PAP Smear										
PSA										
Other tests:										

2. Now that you have charted all of Ms. Davison's blood chemistry results in the flow sheet, compare the results with the document entitled "Garrels—Common Chemistry Panels" located in the Simulations folder of your Evolve course. (*Hint:* Consult your instructor if you need help accessing this document. Notations for normal and abnormal values have been included for tests that are not listed in the table.) On the flow sheet in question 1, place an asterisk (*) after any results that should be given prompt attention.

- Click **Close Chart** when finished to return to the Check Out area.
- Click the exit arrow in the lower right corner of the screen to exit the room.
- On the Summary Menu, click **Return to Map**. Then click **Yes** at the pop-up menu to return to the office map or click **Exit the Program**.

LESSON 25

Medical Microbiology

Patient: Tristan Tsosie

Learning Objectives:

- Discuss the difference between pathogens and nonpathogens.
- Understand the proper procedure for obtaining wound exudate for microbiological testing.
- Identify the correct handling and transportation of a microbiological specimen.
- Discuss the reasons for using appropriate personal protective equipment (PPE) when obtaining microbiological specimens.
- Document the transport of a microbiological specimen in the laboratory log.
- Apply critical thinking skills in answering questions regarding inconsistency in charting examples.

Overview:

This lesson discusses the proper procedure for obtaining specimens for microbiological testing. Tristan Tsosie, an 8-year-old boy with a history of injury to his arm, is now visiting the clinic with a sore throat. You will determine the proper care of Tristan to fulfill the orders of the physician. The patient, who is to have suture removal and a cast check, is accompanied by his sister and another child. During this lesson you should note some inconsistencies; you can comment on these inconsistencies in the Critical Thinking Questions in the lesson.

Important Reminder: When you access a patient's Progress Notes at Mountain View Clinic, first be sure you are in the appropriate room to see the relevant notes.

Exercise 1

 Online Activity—Obtaining a Wound Specimen for Microbiological Testing

 20 minutes

- Sign in to Mountain View Clinic.
- From the patient list, select **Tristan Tsosie**.
- On the office map, click on **Exam Room**. (*Note:* If you want to refresh your memory about this patient, first go to the **Reception** from the office map and review the **Patient Check-In** video. Then return to the office map and click on **Exam Room**.)
- Under the Watch heading, click on **Wound Care** and watch the video.

1. In the video, the medical assistant states that a wound specimen for testing will be obtained. Why is the wound specimen taken from Tristan's arm?

2. Why should the specimen be taken before cleansing the wound?

→ • Click the **X** in the upper right corner to close the video and return to the Exam Room.
- Click on the **Exam Notes** file folder to review the initial documentation of Tristan Tsosie's visit.

3. What tests have been ordered for Tristan?

→ • Click **Finish** to close the Exam Notes and return to the Exam Room.
- Click on **Prepare Room**.

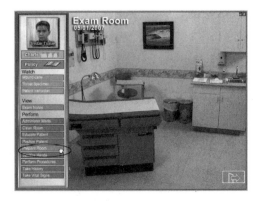

• Add the supplies needed for Tristan's examination by clicking on the supply from the Available Supplies list and clicking **Add Item** to confirm your choice. The items you select will appear in the Selected Supplies box. When you click on an item, a photograph of that item will appear, which can be used for reference as you review your list of supplies. (Note: You can reopen the Exam Notes located in the lower left-hand corner for reference as you make your selections.)

• If you wish to remove a chosen supply, highlight the supply in the Selected Supplies box and click **Remove**.

• Repeat these steps until you are satisfied you have everything you need from the list.

• Once you have made your selections, click **Finish** to return to the Exam Room.

4. Describe the difference between pathogens and nonpathogens. Explain the importance of this difference as it applies to wound care.

5. Indicate whether each one of the following statements is true or false.

a. _____ The wound specimen should be taken from the cleanest area of the wound.

b. _____ Wound specimens should be placed in the transport medium immediately after they are obtained.

c. _____ Wound specimens should be dry for transport so that the chance of cross contamination is reduced.

d. _____ Ideally, wound specimens should be obtained after antibiotic therapy has been initiated.

e. _____ Hands should be sanitized before and after collecting the specimen, even though gloves have been worn.

f. _____ Supplies used in the collection of the wound specimen should be disposed of in the biohazardous waste container.

g. _____ Collection of all wound specimens requires the use of gowns and goggles.

h. _____ Collection of the wound specimen is not complete until documentation has been completed.

i. _____ The amount of time between collecting the specimen and the laboratory processing of the specimen is not important.

6. Describe the means used by the medical assistant and the extern to place Tristan at ease during the procedure of collecting the wound specimen.

Critical Thinking Question

7. Would you have done anything differently if you were the medical assistant taking care of Tristan? (*Hint:* If you need to refresh your memory from an earlier lesson, such as when Tristan was checked in, you may go to the Reception area and review the check-in video.)

 • Click on the **Exam Notes** file folder to read the documentation concerning the wound.

8. The following Progress Notes form is from Tristan's chart; it shows how the wound specimen collection was documented. Compare this documentation against the Exam Notes. Is there any information that could be or should be added to this documentation? Explain.

| 05-01-2007 11:45am | Wound culture obtained, wound cleaned, 7 stitches removed, and new posterior splint reapplied without apparent intolerance. Appears comfortable, no complaints. Fingers pink and warm. QuickVue In-Line One Step Strep A test done; results negative. Wound culture to be sent to QualityLab on 05/02/2007. Given verbal and written instructions on observing for signs of infection, proper splint care, and activity during the healing process. Instructed to have parent call in 2 days with update and to confirm understanding of follow-up care.-- ——*Cathy Wright, CMA* |
| 05-01-2007 12:00pm | Mother contacted and given instructions about required follow-up care.———————————————————— ——*Leah Tran, CMA* |

Critical Thinking Question

9. Assume that the laboratory courier had already picked up the specimens on 5/1/07. What would be the appropriate measures to take to ensure specimen integrity?

Critical Thinking Question

10. How will the medical assistant know the temperature in which to store the specimen until the laboratory courier arrives on the next day?

 • Click **Finish** to close the Exam Notes and return to the Exam Room.
   • Remain in the Exam Room with Tristan Tsosie and continue to the next exercise.

Exercise 2

 Online Activity—Collecting a Throat Specimen for Microbiological Testing

 20 minutes

Note: The Policy Manual does not specify the needed personal protective equipment (PPE) for a professional who is obtaining a throat specimen; it simply states that the Occupational Safety and Health Administration (OSHA) standard precautions should be followed.

1. What PPE should be worn by the medical assistant while obtaining a routine throat specimen? When is it necessary to wear other PPE, and what should be used?

 • Under the Watch heading, click on **Throat Specimen** and watch the video.

2. What did the medical assistant do to ensure that she had Tristan's cooperation?

 • Click the **X** in the upper right corner to close the video and return to the Exam Room.
   • Click the exit arrow in the lower right corner of the screen to exit the room.
   • On the Summary Menu, click on **Look at Your Performance Summary**.
   • Scroll down the Performance Summary to the Prepare Room section and compare your answers with those chosen by the experts.
   • You may save and print the performance summary for your records or to turn it in to your instructor. The icons for saving and printing the Performance Summary are located at the top right corner of the screen.
   • Click **Close** to return to the Summary Menu.
   • On the Summary Menu, click **Return to Map** and select **Yes** at the pop-up menu to return to the office map.

- On the office map, click on **Laboratory**.
- Click on **Collect Specimens** to collect the specimens that need to be tested for Tristan Tsosie.

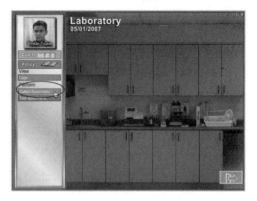

- Use the checkboxes to select the specimens that need to be collected for Tristan's visit. (*Hint:* If you wish to review the notes for this visit, click on **Charts** in the Room Menu, click on the **Patient Medical Information** tab and select **1-Progress Notes**.)
- Click **Next**.
- A series of questions will be asked for each test you selected. Answer all the questions related to each test, using the checkboxes and radio buttons provided. (*Hint:* The Policy Manual can be opened at any time for reference as you answer the questions.)
- Click **Finish** to return to the Laboratory.
- Click on **Charts** to open the patient's medical record.
- Click on the **Patient Medical Information** tab and select **1-Progress Notes** from the drop-down menu.
- Make a notation of the date that the Progress Notes indicate the specimen was sent to QualityLab for analysis.

3. What are the results of the strep test that was processed using the specimen?

4. Was the documentation correct for the testing performed? Explain your answer.

5. When you are obtaining a throat specimen for testing, what is the most appropriate site for collection?

Critical Thinking Question

6. Why would it be advantageous to use two sterile swabs when collecting a specimen? In what situation(s) do you think a specimen would likely be sent to an outside laboratory?

7. Why is it important that the inside of the mouth not be touched while the throat specimen is being obtained?

→ • Click on the **Diagnostic Tests** tab and select **3-Laboratory Requisition Form** from the drop-down menu.
 • Review the Laboratory Requisition for accuracy and completeness.

8. Is the Laboratory Requisition complete and correct? If not, describe any errors and explain what would need to be done to correct them.

9. What insurance information is to be provided with the Laboratory Requisition?

→ • Click **Close Chart** when finished to return to the Laboratory.
 • Click on the **Lab Log Binder** to view the log of tests recently performed in the laboratory.

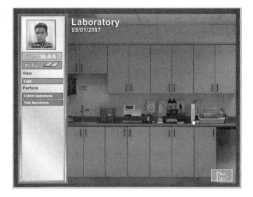

10. Are all of the tests properly logged for quality control and for following the results of the tests?

11. Earlier in the lesson, what did the documentation in the Exam Room say about the date of the transport of the culture to the reference laboratory?

12. Does your answer to question 11 differ from what was documented in the Progress Notes when you accessed them from the Laboratory? If so, what did the Laboratory Progress Notes indicate?

Critical Thinking Question

13. Why would it be important to pick up on discrepancies in charting concerning what happens in the medical office? Does it really matter which date is listed for the transport of the culture, as addressed in the previous questions?

14. On the following blank log, document the transport of the wound specimen to the laboratory using the 05/01/07 date. Use the initials CLW as the person who collected the specimen.

Requisition Number	Date of Specimen Collection	Patient Name	Laboratory Test	Processing Lab	Initials: Specimen Collection	Date of Results Return	Initials: Results Return

 • Click **Finish** to close the log and return to the Laboratory.
- Click the exit arrow in the lower right corner of the screen to exit the room.
- On the Summary Menu, click on **Look at Your Performance Summary**.
- Scroll down the Performance Summary to the appropriate section and compare your answers with those chosen by the experts.
- You may save and print the Performance Summary for your records or turn it in to your instructor. The icons for saving and printing the Performance Summary are located at the top right corner of the screen.
- Click **Close** to return to the Summary Menu.
- On the Summary Menu, click **Return to Map**, then click **Yes** at the pop-up menu to return to the office map or click **Exit the Program**.

The Medical Record

Patients: Renee Anderson, Tristan Tsosie

Learning Objectives:

- Understand the importance of correctly organizing a patient's medical information.
- Identify and describe the forms found in a medical record.
- Apply principles of medical record organization to choose forms that would be needed when preparing a new patient's medical record.
- Determine whether forms need to be added to the medical record for an established patient.
- Describe the appropriate care of a damaged medical record.
- Distinguish among reports for appropriate filing in the medical record.
- Identify the advantages and disadvantages of using an electronic medical record (EMR) or electronic health record (EHR) in the medical office.
- Recognize the correct meaning of common abbreviations used in the medical record.

Overview:

This lesson explores the importance of correctly preparing a patient's medical record and placing reports that are received in the appropriate section of the chart. Because the medical record is a legal document that shows the chronological care of the patient, this document must be correctly organized to ensure that information can be located as needed. Incorrectly organized charts not only cause frustration but also decrease the efficiency of the medical practice. You will organize a medical record for a new patient. For an established patient, you will ensure that information received from other sources has been properly organized and that the information is readily available when the patient arrives for an appointment. You will also review reports and then determine in what area of the chart each report should be filed. In addition, you will define or identify definitions for important abbreviations used in the medical record.

Exercise 1

Online Activity—Organizing a Medical Record for a New Patient

30 minutes

- Sign in to Mountain View Clinic.
- From the patient list, select **Renee Anderson**.
- On the office map, click on **Reception**.
- Click on **Policy** to open the office Policy Manual.
- Type "job descriptions" in the search bar and click on the magnifying glass.
- Scroll down to read the duties assigned to the various types of medical assistants in the office.

1. At Mountain View Clinic, the Policy Manual states that the _____ medical assistant is responsible for preparing and organizing the medical record.

Critical Thinking Question

2. Why is it so important for the administrative medical assistant to place the necessary forms in a medical record for a new patient immediately after the patient has checked in at the registration desk?

• Click **Close Manual** to return to the Reception area.

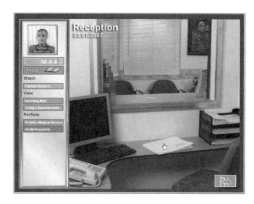

• Click on the **Medical Record** on the counter to assemble a chart for Renee Anderson's visit.

• Click on the **Perform** button next to Assemble Medical Record.

• The Patient Information tab is automatically chosen as the starting point when you access the Assemble Medical Record screen.

• Add forms needed in the Patient Information tab by clicking on the forms from the Forms Available list and then clicking **Add** to confirm your choice. The forms you select will appear under the tabs at the bottom of the screen.

• When you have completed the Patient Information section, continue adding forms to any additional appropriate tabs in the patient's medical record. To select a new tab, either click on the tab on the medical record or use the drop-down menu on the right.

• If you wish to remove a chosen form, highlight the form and click **Remove** at the bottom of the screen.

3. The form that contains the patient's demographic and billing information is the

   _____.

4. The form in the medical record that contains subjective information about the patient's

   illnesses in the past is the _____.

5. The document that explains to patients how their health information will be used and

   protected by the medical office is the _____.

6. The form that allows the physician to update the medical record with new information when

   the patient visits or telephones the office is the _____
   form.

 • When you are satisfied that you have selected all the necessary forms and put them in the correct tab sections, click **Finish** to close the chart and return to the Reception area.

• While registering the patient, the administrative medical assistant will also ask whether the patient has insurance coverage.

• Click on the **Insurance Card** on the counter to obtain Renee Anderson's insurance information.

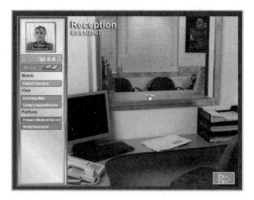

- Identify the appropriate question to ask Ms. Anderson regarding her insurance and click on **Ask**.
- Use the checkboxes to select which procedures are needed to verify the patient's insurance. (*Note:* If you need help, you can open the relevant sections of the patient's chart for reference as you make your selections.)
- Click **Finish** to return to the Reception area.
- Click the exit arrow in the lower right corner of the screen to exit the Reception area.
- On the Summary Menu, click on **Look at Your Performance Summary**.
- Scroll down the **Performance Summary** to the Patient Records section and the Verify Insurance section and compare your answers with those chosen by the experts.
- You may save and print the Performance Summary for your records or turn it in to your instructor. The icons for saving and printing the Performance Summary are located at the top right corner of the screen.
- Click **Close** to return to the Summary Menu.
- On the Summary Menu, click **Return to Map** and select **Yes** at the pop-up menu to return to the office map.

Exercise 2

Online Activity—Adding to the Medical Record of an Established Patient

 20 minutes

- From the patient list, select **Tristan Tsosie**.
- On the office map, click on **Reception**.
- Click on **Charts** to open the patient's medical record.
- Click on the **Hospitalization** tab and select **1-ED Record** (Emergency Department Record) from the drop-down menu.

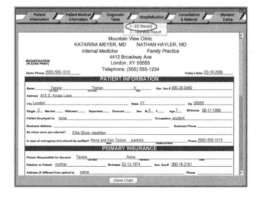

• Read the ED Record to decide what other forms should be available for the physician for this office visit and to determine whether Tristan is following the orders of the physician who saw him in the emergency department. Think about which procedures the patient had while in the emergency department and which of those would have a report to be filed in his chart. Then look under other tabs of the chart to see whether you can find additional reports that you would also need to have available for the physician.

• Click **Close Chart** when finished to return to the Reception area.

• Click on the **Medical Record** to review and add forms to Tristan Tsosie's chart for this visit.

• Click on the **Perform** button next to Review and Update Medical Records.

• The Patient Information tab is automatically chosen as the starting point when you access the Assemble Medical Record screen.

• Review the forms listed under the Patient Information tab. Add any forms that are missing from the Patient Information tab by clicking on the forms from the Forms Available list and then clicking **Add** to confirm your choice. The forms you select will appear under the tabs at the bottom of the screen.

• When you have completed the Patient Information section, continue reviewing and adding forms to other appropriate tabs in Tristan Tsosie's medical record. To select a new tab, either click on the tab on the medical record itself or use the drop-down menu on the right.

• If you wish to remove a chosen form, highlight the form in the tab and click **Remove** at the bottom of the screen.

• When you are satisfied that you have selected all the necessary forms and put them in the correct tab sections, click **Finish** to close the chart and return to the Reception area.

• Go back and read the notes from the ED Record under the Hospitalization tab and the Consultation Notes under the Consultation and Referral tab, making note of the patient instructions for follow-up.

1. According to the ED Record, where was Tristan instructed to follow up?

2. According to the Consultation Notes, when was Tristan supposed to follow up with the physician? (*Note:* Specify in number of days.)

Critical Thinking Question

3. If a patient folder is old, torn, or simply worn, what should the medical assistant do?

• Click the exit arrow in the lower right corner of the screen to exit the Reception area.

• On the Summary Menu, click on **Look at Your Performance Summary**.

• Scroll down the Performance Summary to the Patient Records section and compare your answers with those chosen by the experts.

• You may save and print the performance summary for your records or turn it in to your instructor. The icons for saving and printing the Performance Summary are located at the top right corner of the screen.

• Click **Close** to return to the Summary Menu.

• On the Summary Menu, click **Return to Map** and select **Yes** at the pop-up menu to return to the office map or click **Exit the Program**.

Exercise 3

Writing Activity—Medical Record Categorizing

20 minutes

1. Most of the records that are filed in a patient's medical record belong to one of the following categories:

   • Consent Documents
   • Diagnostic Procedure Documents
   • Hospital Documents
   • Medical Office Administrative Documents
   • Medical Office Clinical Documents
   • Problem-Oriented Records
   • Therapeutic Service Documents

   Review the records on the pages that follow. In the blank above each record, write the name of the category in which it belongs. (*Note:* You will use some categories more than once.)

a. _____

HISTORY AND PHYSICAL
ST. MERCY HOSPITAL

Patient Name: _Carol Jacobs_   Room #: _215_

Physician: _Charles Thomas, MD_   Hospital #: _5422_

Admission Date: _12/14/12_

CHIEF COMPLAINT: Chest pain

HISTORY OF PRESENT ILLNESS: Patient is an 85-year-old female complaining of chest pain. Patient was found to have abnormal cardiac enzymes in the Emergency Room consistent with acute myocardial infarction. Patient denied any pain radiating; however, she did complain of left-sided chest pain and lower back pain. Patient did not admit to any shortness of breath, nausea, or diaphoresis.

MEDICATIONS: Lasix, Darvocet-N 100, Lisinopril, Lopressor, Glynase, Relafen, Cytotec, and Micro K.

ALLERGIES: No drug allergies known.

PAST MEDICAL HISTORY: Significant for congestive heart failure, chronic obstructive pulmonary disease, diabetes mellitus type 2, coronary atherosclerosis, hypertension, and osteoporosis.

SOCIAL HISTORY: Not a drinker and not a smoker. Patient resides in a nursing home.

PHYSICAL EXAMINATION:

General: Patient is in acute distress. She is obese.

HEENT: She has 2 centimeters jugular venous distention. Pupils are equal and reactive to light and accommodation. No evidence of scleral or conjunctival icterus.

Chest: +2 bibasilar rales.

Heart: Regular rate and rhythm. +2/6 systolic ejection murmur in the left sternal border.

Abdomen: Soft, nontender, no splenomegaly and no hepatomegaly and positive bowel sounds.

Extremities: No evidence of edema or deep venous thrombosis.

Neurological: Cranial nerves II through XII grossly intact.

IMPRESSIONS: Congestive heart failure
Rule out myocardial infarction

Charles Thomas, MD

Charles Thomas, MD

b. _____

COLLEGE HOSPITAL
4567 BROAD AVENUE
WOODLAND HILLS, MD 21532

RADIOLOGY REPORT

Examination Date:	June 14, 2012	Patient:	Rose Baker
Date Reported:	June 14, 2012	X-ray No.:	43200
Physician:	Harold B. Cooper, M.D.	Age:	19
Examination:	PA Chest, Abdomen	Hospital No.:	80-32-11

FINDINGS

PA CHEST: Upright PA view of chest shows the lung fields are clear, without evidence of an active process. Heart size is normal. There is no evidence of pneumoperitoneum.

IMPRESSION: NEGATIVE CHEST

ABDOMEN: Flat and upright views of the abdomen show a normal gas pattern without evidence of obstruction or ileus. There are no calcifications or abnormal masses noted.

IMPRESSION: NEGATIVE STUDY

RADIOLOGIST: *Marian B. Skinner*

Marian B. Skinner, MD

c. _____

DISCHARGE SUMMARY

Brennan, Susan
97-32-11
June 18, 2012

ADMISSION DATE: June 14, 2012   **DISCHARGE DATE:** June 16, 2012

HISTORY OF PRESENT ILLNESS:
This 19-year-old female, nulligravida, was admitted to the hospital on June 14, 2012, with fever of 102°, left lower quadrant pain, vaginal discharge, constipation, and a tender left adnexal mass. Her past history and family history were unremarkable. Present pain had started two to three weeks prior to admission. Her periods were irregular, with latest period starting on May 30, 2012, and lasting for six days. She had taken contraceptive pills in the past but had stopped because she was not sexually active.

PHYSICAL EXAMINATION:
She appeared well developed and well nourished, and in mild distress. The only positive physical findings were limited to the abdomen and pelvis. Her abdomen was mildly distended, and it was tender, especially in the left lower quadrant. At pelvic examination, her cervix was tender on motion, and the uterus was of normal size, retroverted, and somewhat fixed. There was a tender cystic mass about 4-5 cm in the left adnexa. Rectal examination was negative.

PROVISIONAL DIAGNOSIS:
1. Probable pelvic inflammatory disease (PID).
2. Rule out ectopic pregnancy.

LABORATORY DATA ON ADMISSION:
Hgb 10.8, Hct 36.5, WBC 8,100 with 80 segs and 18 lymphs. Sedimentation rate 100 mm in one hour. Sickle cell prep+ (turned out to be a trait). Urinalysis normal. Electrolytes normal. SMA-12 normal. Chest x-ray negative, 2-hour UCG negative.

HOSPITAL COURSE AND TREATMENT:
Initially, she was given cephalothin 2 gm IV q6h, and kanamycin 0.5 gm IM bid. Over the next two days the patient's condition improved. Her pain decreased and her temperature came down to normal in the morning and spiked to 101° in the evening. Repeat CBC showed Hgb 9.8, Hct 33.5. The pregnancy test was negative. She was discharged on June 16, 2012 in good condition. She will be seen in the office in one week.

DISCHARGE DIAGNOSIS:
Pelvic inflammatory disease.

Harold B. Cooper, MD
Harold B. Cooper, MD

d. _____

EMERGENCY DEPARTMENT REPORT
CAMDEN CLARK HOSPITAL

Name: _John Larimer_ DOB: _2/2/72_

ER Physician: _John Parsons, MD_ Date: _7/7/12_

ER Number: _07398_

Physician: _James Woods, MD_

NATURE OF ILLNESS/INJURY: This 40-year-old male presents to the Emergency Department complaining of a laceration of the sole of his right foot. Patient cut his foot on a rock 2 days ago and thinks he might have an infection now. Patient also complains of coughing over the past several days.

PHYSICAL EXAMINATION: Temperature 97.4, Pulse 76, Respirations 20, Blood Pressure 120/70. Patient is alert and oriented and is in no acute distress. ENT is normal. Lungs show diffuse rhonchi without crackles or wheezing. Heart has a regular rate and rhythm. Right great toe with marked tenderness with edema and erythema and heat.

DIAGNOSIS: Asthmatic Bronchitis
Cellulitis, right foot first MTP

TREATMENT: PCMX scrub to right foot. Bacitracin dressing. Tetanus Diphtheria 0.5 cc IM. Biaxin 500 mg bid x 10 days. Guaifenesin with codeine 2 tsp q4h prn. Entex LA,1 bid prn. Debridement of skin flap.

PATIENT INSTRUCTIONS: Patient to follow up with family doctor in 7 days. Discussed bronchospasms with the patient.

Jam— Woods, MD
_____
James Woods, MD

e. _____

(Attach label or complete blanks.)

First name: _____ Last name: _____

Date of Birth: _____ Month _____ Day _____ Year

Account Number: _____

Procedure Consent Form

I, _____ , hereby consent to have

Dr. _____ perform _____

I have been fully informed of the following by my physician:

1. The nature of my condition
2. The nature and purpose of the procedure
3. An explanation of risks involved with the procedure
4. Alternative treatments or procedures available
5. The likely results of the procedure
6. The risks involved with declining or delaying the procedure

My physician has offered to answer all questions concerning the proposed procedure.

I am aware that the practice of medicine and surgery is not an exact science, and I acknowledge that no guarantees have been made to me about the results of the procedure.

Patient _____ Date _____
(or guardian and relationship)

Witnessed _____ Date _____

f. _____

Date	**Time**	**Problem Number**	**FORMAT:** **Problem Number and TITLE:** S = Subjective O = Objective A = Assessment P = Plan			

PROBLEM ORIENTED - PROGRESS NOTES

Date	Time	Problem Number	FORMAT: Problem Number and TITLE: S = Subjective O = Objective A = Assessment P = Plan
11/15/12	9:30 AM	1	S: Mother states that her child has had a runny nose and her throat has been
			sore for 2 days.
			O: Vital signs: T 98.8 P 96 R 24
			Weight: 42 lb.
			General: alert and active. HEENT: sclera clear. TMs negative. Positive clear
			rhinorrhea. Pharynx benign. Heart: regular without murmur.
			Lungs: clear to auscultation and percussion. Abdomen: negative tenderness.
			Positive bowel x 4. GU: negative. Neuro: good tone.
			A: Upper respiratory tract infection.
			P: 1. A prescription for Rondec DM, 1/2 tsp q6h prn cough and congestion.
			2. Instructed mother to contact office if child does not improve.

NAME-Last	First	Middle	Attending Physician	Record No.	Room/Bed
Michaels	Jessica	L	Frank Edwards, MD	1	24

Form 6612/SS © 2010/SS, Des Moines, IA 50306 (800) 247-2343 www.BriggsCorp.com
PRINTED IN U.S.A.

PROBLEM ORIENTED - PROGRESS NOTES

g. _____

OPERATIVE REPORT
ST. MARY'S HOSPITAL

Name: Natalie Boyer

Hospital #: 291734   Room #: OP

Surgeon: Paul Cain, M.D.   Date of Surgery: 1/6/12

Assistants: N/A   Anesthesia: General

Anesthesiologist: John Adams, M.D.

PRE-OP DIAGNOSIS: Abnormal Pap test with history of cervical carcinoma.

POST-OP DIAGNOSIS: Same and awaiting path report.

PROCEDURE: D&C, laser cone of the cervix.

The patient to the operating room, lithotomy position, perineum and vagina were prepped, and moist sterile drape was used. Laser precautions all in place. Bimanual examination revealed a uterus enlarged with a second-degree uterine prolapse. The cervix was dilated. Uterus sounded to around 9 cm. The endocervical canal was dilated and D&C was performed with tissue recovered and submitted to Pathology. The cervix was stained with iodine, and the nonstaining area was identified. The laser was brought in, 50 watts of current were used to remove laser cone, and we submitted that to Pathology. We then vaporized beyond the margins of the cone, 3-4 mm to a depth of 4-5 mm. Hemostasis was adequate. We placed 0 Vicryl figure-of-eight sutures at the 3 and the 9 o'clock positions in the cervix, and then we put Monsel solution on the cervix. Hemostasis adequate. Sponge and needle counts correct times two. The patient tolerated the procedure well, and she returned to the recovery room in stable condition. She will be discharged home when awake and stable on Cipro 250 mg twice a day for a week, Darvocet-N 100, #20 as needed for pain. If she continues to have abnormal Pap tests, we will probably want to do a vaginal hysterectomy.

SURGEON: _Paul Cain, MD_

Paul Cain, MD

h. _____

HAROLD B. COOPER, M.D.
6000 MAIN STREET
VENTURA, CA 93003

June 15, 2012

John F. Millstone, M.D.
5302 Main Street
Ventura, CA 93003

Dear Dr. Millstone:

RE: Elaine J. Silverman

This 69-year-old woman was seen at your request. The patient was admitted to the hospital yesterday because of chills, fever, and abdominal and back pain.

REVIEW OF HEALTH HISTORY: The history has been reviewed. A prominent feature of the history is the presence of intermittent, severe, shaking chills for four days with associated left lower back pain, left lower quadrant abdominal pain, and fever to as high as 103 or 104 degrees. The patient has had hypertension for a number of years and has been managed quite well with Aldomet 250 mg twice a day.

PHYSICAL EXAMINATION: On examination her temperature at this time is 100.6 degrees. The pulse is 110 and regular. Blood pressure is 190/100. The patient has partial bilateral iridectomies, the result of previous cataract surgery. Otherwise, the head and neck are not remarkable. Lung fields are clear throughout. The heart reveals a regular tachycardia, and heart sounds are of good quality. No murmurs are heard, and there is no gallop rhythm present. The abdomen is soft. There is no spasm or guarding. A well-healed surgical scar is present in the right flank area. There is considerable tenderness in the left lower quadrant of the left mid abdomen, but as noted, there is no spasm or guarding present. Bowel sounds are present. Peristaltic rushes are noted, and the bowel sounds are slightly high pitched. The extremities are unremarkable.

IMPRESSIONS: I believe the patient has acute diverticulitis. She may have some irritation of the left ureter in view of the findings on the urinalysis. She appears to be responding to therapy at this time in that her temperature is coming down and there has been a slight reduction in the leukocytosis from yesterday.

RECOMMENDATIONS: I agree with the present program of therapy, and the only suggestion would be to possibly increase the dose of gentamicin to 60 mg q8h, rather than the 40 mg q8h that she is now receiving.

Thank you for asking me to see this patient in consultation.

Sincerely,

Harold B. Cooper

Harold B. Cooper, M.D.

mtf

i. _____

PHYSICAL THERAPY EVALUATION

OBJECTIVE DATA TESTS AND SCALES PRINTED ON REVERSE.

DATE OF SERVICE 9 / 23 / 12

HOMEBOUND REASON: ☐ Needs assistance for all activities   ☐ Residual weakness
☐ Requires assistance to ambulate   ☐ Confusion, unable to go out of home alone
☐ Unable to safely leave home unassisted   ☐ Severe SOB, SOB upon exertion
☐ Dependent upon adaptive device(s)   ☐ Medical restrictions
☐ Other (specify)_____

SOC DATE 9 / 23 / 12

[If Initial Evaluation, complete Physical Therapy Care Plan]

PERTINENT BACKGROUND INFORMATION

OTHER DISCIPLINES PROVIDING CARE: ☐ SN ☐ OT ☐ ST ☐ MSW ☐ Aide

MEDICAL HISTORY

☐ Hypertension   ☐ Cancer
☐ Cardiac   ☐ Infection
☐ Diabetes   ☐ Immunosuppressed
☐ Respiratory   ☐ Open wound
☐ Osteoporosis   ☐ Falls with injury
☐ Fractures   ☐ Falls without injury
☐ Other (specify)_____

REASON FOR EVALUATION (Diagnosis / Problem)

Hx Ⓛ knee pain x 5 yrs, little relief č PT

LIVING SITUATION

☒ Capable ☐ Able ☐ Willing caregiver available
☐ Limited caregiver support (ability/willingness)
☐ No caregiver available
HOME SAFETY BARRIERS:
☐ Clutter ☐ Throw rugs ☐ Bath bench/equipment ☐ Needs grab bar
☐ Needs railings ☐ Steps (number/condition)
☐ Other (specify)_____

PRIOR LEVEL OF FUNCTION

ADLs:
☒ Independent ☐ Needed assistance ☐ Unable
Equipment used:_____

IN-HOME MOBILITY (gait or wheelchair/scooter):
☒ Independent ☐ Needed assistance ☐ Unable
Equipment used:_____

COMMUNITY MOBILITY (gait or wheelchair/scooter):
☐ Independent ☐ Needed assistance ☐ Unable
Equipment used:_____

BEHAVIOR / MENTAL STATUS

☒ Alert ☐ Oriented ☐ Cooperative ☐ Confused ☐ Memory deficits
☐ Impaired judgement ☐ Other (specify)_____

VITAL SIGNS / CURRENT STATUS

Blood Pressure:_____
Temperature:_____
Pulse:_____
Respirations:_____
O₂ saturation _____% (when ordered): ☐ at rest ☐ with activity
Skin:_____
Edema:_____
Vision: glasses
Sensation:_____
Communication:_____
Hearing:_____
Posture:_____
Endurance:_____

PAIN

INTENSITY: 0 1 2 3 4 ⑤ 6 7 8 9 10
LOCATION:_____
AGGRAVATING FACTORS:_____

RELIEVING FACTORS:_____

BEST PAIN GETS: 2   **WORST PAIN GETS:** 8
ACCEPTABLE LEVEL OF PAIN:_____
CURRENT LEVEL OF PAIN:_____
IMPACT ON THERAPY POC? ☐ None ☐ (describe)_____

PATIENT NAME – Last, First, Middle Initial
Johnson, Thomas, J.

ID#

PHYSICAL THERAPY EVALUATION
☐ Continued on Reverse

j. _____

RELEASE OF MEDICAL INFORMATION

All information contained in the medical record is confidential, and the release of information is closely controlled. A properly completed and signed authorization form is required for the release of the following information.

PATIENT INFORMATION

Patient Name _____

Address _____ Social Security # _____

City _____ State _____ ZIP _____ Birth date ____/____/____

Phone (Home) _____ Work _____

RELEASE FROM:

Name _____

Address _____

City _____ State _____ ZIP _____

RELEASE TO:

Name _____

Address _____

City _____ State _____ ZIP _____

INFORMATION TO BE RELEASED:

1. GENERAL RELEASE:

____ Entire Medical Record (excluding protected information)
____ Hospital Records only (specify) _____
____ Lab Results only (specify) _____
____ X-ray Reports only (specify) _____
____ Other Records (specify) _____

2. INFORMATION PROTECTED BY STATE/FEDERAL LAW:
If indicated below, I hereby authorize the disclosure and release of information regarding:

____ Drug Abuse Diagnosis/Treatment
____ Alcoholism Diagnosis/Treatment
____ Mental Health Diagnosis/Treatment
____ Sexually Transmitted Disease

PURPOSE/NEED FOR INFORMATION:

____ Taking records to another doctor
____ Moving
____ Legal purposes
____ Insurance purposes
____ Worker's Compensation
____ Other/Explain: _____

METHOD OF RELEASE:

____ US Mail

____ Fax

____ Telephone

____ To Patient

PATIENT AUTHORIZATION TO RELEASE INFORMATION:

Authorization is valid for 60 days only from the date of my signature. I reserve the right to revoke this authorization at any time prior to 60 days (except for action that has already been taken) by notifying the medical office in writing.

I understand that my records are protected under HIPAA (Health Insurance Portability and Accountability Act) Standards for Privacy of Individually Identifiable Information (45 CFR Parts 160 and 164) unless otherwise permitted by federal law. Any information released or received shall not be further relayed to any other facility or person without my written authorization. I also understand that such information will not be given, sold, transferred, or in any way relayed to any other person or party not specified above without my further written authorization.

I hereby grant authorization to release the information listed above. I certify that this request has been made voluntarily and that the information given above is accurate to the best of my knowledge.

_____   _____
Signature of Patient/Legally Responsible Party   Date

_____   _____
Witness Signature   Date

OFFICE USE ONLY

Information indicated above released on _____
                                        Date

Explanation of information released: _____

_____

Signature and credentials of individual releasing information: _____

k. _____

PATIENT INFORMATION	CONFIDENTIAL		File no. 10140

PATIENT INFORMATION   **CONFIDENTIAL**

File no. 10140
Date 11-21-12

(PLEASE PRINT)

Name Carol   H   Jones   Birth date 1-20-68   Home phone 740-555-1248
     First   Middle   Last

Address 743 Evergreen Terrace   City Springfield   State OH   ZIP 12345

Check appropriate box: ☐ Minor ☐ Single ☒ Married ☐ Divorced ☐ Widowed ☐ Separated   Gender: ☐ Male ☒ Female

Employer Rockford, Inc.   Work phone 740-555-1234

Business address 1 Rockford Place   City Shelbyville   State OH   ZIP 21346

Spouse or parent's name John Jones   Employer Self-emp.   Work phone 740-555-8654

If patient is a student, name of school/college N/A   City _____ State _____

Whom may we thank for referring you? Henry Peterson, MD

Person to contact in case of emergency John Jones   Phone 740-555-1248

RESPONSIBLE PARTY

Name of person responsible for this account Carol Jones   Relationship to patient Self

Address 743 Evergreen Terrace   City Springfield   State OH   ZIP 12345   Home phone 740-555-1248

Employer Rockford, Inc.   Work phone 740-555-1234

Is this person currently a patient in our office?   ☒ Yes   ☐ No

INSURANCE INFORMATION

Name of insured Carol Jones   Relationship to patient Self

Birth date 1-20-68   Social Security number 123-45-6789   Date employed 5-1-93

Name of employer Rockford, Inc.   Work phone 740-555-1234

Address of employer 1 Rockford Place   City Shelbyville   State OH   ZIP 21346

Insurance company Anthem BC/BS   Group number 51045

Insurance company address 521 Anthem Drive   City New Haberville   State OH   ZIP 21436

DO YOU HAVE ANY ADDITIONAL INSURANCE? ☐ YES ☒ NO   IF YES, COMPLETE THE FOLLOWING:

Name of insured _____   Relationship to patient _____

Birth date _____   Social Security number _____   Date employed _____

Name of employer _____   Work phone _____

Address of employer _____   City _____ State _____ ZIP _____

Insurance company _____   Group number _____

Insurance company address _____   City _____ State _____ ZIP _____

X _Carol Jones_

SIGNATURE OF PATIENT OR PARENT IF MINOR

1. _____

DIAGNOSTIC IMAGING REPORT

Mt. Carmel Hospital,
Columbus, OH 43201

DATE REQUESTED	DATE TO BE DONE	TODAY'S DATE	DATE OF BIRTH
6/6/2012	6/10/2012	6/10/2012	8/19/1949

☐ WHEELCHAIR   ☐ PORTABLE   ☒ AMBULATORY   ☐ CART

PATIENT:
Vera Ruth

INSURANCE:
Industrial

SEX	ROOM NO.	RESPONSIBLE PERSON OR EMPLOYER
F	OP	J.B. Warren, Inc.

RADIOLOGIST
Richard W. Adams, MD

ATTENDING PHYSICIAN
Christopher Robb, MD

NURSE

CLINICAL INFORMATION AND PROVISIONAL DIAGNOSIS

Back injury

EXAMINATION REQUESTED (PINPOINT AREA OF CONCERN IF POSSIBLE)
CT LUMBAR SPINE

TECHNIQUE:

CT of the lumbar spine without contrast was performed from L-3 through S-1.

FINDINGS:

The L3-4 level appears satisfactory without evidence of osseous proliferation or disc protrusion.

At the L4-5 level there is some increased density at the disc level, which may be more prominent on the left. This is partially obscured due to facet artifact crossing obliquely.

There does appear to be some retention of epidural fat plane. This, however, may represent left-sided disc bulge or protrusion with the appropriate corresponding clinical appearance. Osseous variation at this level is not identified.

At the L5-S1 level, significant variation is not apparent.

IMPRESSION:

Variation at the L4-5 level on the left, which may represent annular disc bulge or perhaps protrusion on the left. However, confirmation with myelography and/or Ampaque enhanced computed tomography of the lumbar spine should be suggested prior to any surgical intervention.

Richard W. Adams, MD

Richard W. Adams, MD

m._____

COLLEGE HOSPITAL
4567 BROAD AVENUE
WOODLAND HILLS, MD 21532

PATHOLOGY REPORT

Date:	June 20, 2012	Pathology No.:	430211
Patient:	Molly Ramsdale	Room No.:	1308
Physician:	Harold B. Cooper, M.D.		
Specimen Submitted:	Tumor, right axilla		

FINDINGS

GROSS DESCRIPTION: Specimen A consists of an oval mass of yellow fibroadipose tissue measuring 4 x 3 x 2 cm. On cut section, there are some small, soft, pliable areas of gray apparent lymph node alternating with adipose tissue. A frozen section consultation at time of surgery was delivered as NO EVIDENCE OF MALIGNANCY on frozen section, to await permanent section for final diagnosis. Majority of the specimen will be submitted for microscopic examination.

Specimen B consists of an oval mass of yellow soft tissue measuring 2.5 x 2.5 x 1.5 cm. On cut section, there is a thin rim of pink to tan-brown lymphatic tissue and the mid portion appears to be adipose tissue. A pathological consultation at time of surgery was delivered as no suspicious areas noted and to await permanent sections for final diagnosis. The entire specimen will be submitted for microscopic examination.

MICROSCOPIC DESCRIPTION: Specimen A sections show fibroadipose tissue and nine fragments of lymph nodes. The lymph nodes show areas with prominent germinal centers and moderate sinus histiocytosis. There appears to be some increased vascularity and reactive endothelial cells seen. There is no evidence of malignancy.

Specimen B sections show adipose tissue and 5 lymph node fragments. These 5 portions of lymph nodes show reactive changes including sinus histiocytosis. There is no evidence of malignancy.

DIAGNOSIS: A & B: TUMOR, RIGHT AXILLA: SHOWING 14 LYMPH NODE FRAGMENTS WITH REACTIVE CHANGES AND NO EVIDENCE OF MALIGNANCY.

Stanley T. Nason, MD

Stanley T. Nason, MD

n. _____

PATIENT RECORD									

Name: Morani, Betty
Number: ____ Blood Type: A+
ALLERGIES/SENSITIVITY: Codeine, Sulfa

Prob. No.	Date	PROBLEM DESCRIPTION	Date Resolved	Index	Prob. No.	Date	PROBLEM DESCRIPTION	Date Resolved	Index
1	10/05	Hypertension - essential		✓					
2	10/05	Diabetes mellitus (mild)		✓					
3	1/08	L. Retinopathy	see below						
4	4/2012	Atherosclerosis with cerebral vascular insuffic.							
5	4/2012	Hearing loss							
6	1/2012	HBP Non-compliance	2/12						
3	1/2012	Bilat. Grade II Retinopathy							

Prob. No.	CONTINUING MEDICATIONS	Start	Stop	Prob. No.	CONTINUING MEDICATIONS	Start	Stop
1	Sinoserp 1 mg. b.i.d.	10/05	10/09				
2	Orinase 0.5 gm. daily	10/05	10/09				
1	Hydrodiuril 50 mg. A.M.	10/05					
2	1500 cal. diet low Na hi K	2/2012					

Periodic Health Examination	Dates	1/04	4/06	2/08	1/10					

o. _____

2. The abbreviations below are used frequently in patient medical records. Match each abbreviation with its meaning.

Abbreviation	Meaning
_____ abd	a. Twice a day
_____ AP	b. Immediately
_____ CC	c. Abdomen
_____ LMP	d. By mouth
_____ DOB	e. Without
_____ N/C	f. Four times a day
_____ NB	g. Apical pulse
_____ qid	h. By or through
_____ po	i. Last menstrual period
_____ w/o	j. Newborn
_____ STAT	k. No complaints
_____ per	l. At bedtime
_____ bid	m. Chief complaint
_____ hs	n. Date of birth

Exercise 4

 Writing Activity—Electronic Medical Record and Electronic Health Records: Internet Research

 10 minutes

1. Patient records can be created and accessed in hard-copy (paper) form or as a digital (electronic) record. How do paper medical records differ from those in an electronic medical record (EMR) or an electronic health record (EHR)?

2. List three advantages of an electronic record system.

3. List three disadvantages of an electronic record system.

4. When a medical office converts from a paper record system to an electronic record system how are the records transferred?

Obtaining and Documenting a Health History

Reading Assignment: Chapter 5—The Physical Examination
- Assessment of the Patient

Chapter 36—The Medical Record
- Taking a Health History
- Charting in the Medical Record

Patients: Kevin McKinzie, Hu Huang, Tristan Tsosie, Wilson Metcalf

Learning Objectives:

- State the need for a health history.
- Describe the components of the health history and the importance of each.
- State the questions that should be included during a health history.
- Indicate the accurate method of documenting a health history in a medical record.
- Demonstrate accurate written communication skills.
- Describe the correct documentation of the health history in the Progress Notes.
- Explain the difference between signs and symptoms.
- Differentiate between objective and subjective symptoms.
- Explain the need for confidentiality when obtaining a health history.

Overview:

In this lesson you will learn about the importance of obtaining an accurate health history and how this information can affect patient care. You will review the health histories of several patients and learn about the need for accurate documentation regarding a patient's medical and social histories.

Copyright © 2013, 2009 by Saunders, an imprint of Elsevier Inc. All rights reserved.

Exercise 1

Writing Activity—Background for Obtaining a Health History

30 minutes

1. What components should be included when you obtain a health history?

2. When obtaining a patient's past medical history, why is it important that the medical assistant review this information with the patient rather than just rely on what the patient writes on the form?

3. Why would the physician need to know any previous surgical procedures a patient has undergone and where these procedures were performed?

4. What is included in a social history?

5. Why is it important to include educational background in a medical history?

6. Why are environmental factors important to include in a medical history?

7. Define *chief complaint*.

8. What four questions should the patient be asked to obtain an accurate chief complaint for documentation?

9. An expansion of the chief complaint occurs in the section of the health history called the

   _____.

10. Indicate whether each of the following statements is true or false.

   a. _____ The chief complaint should be detailed and written in as many words as needed to convey the idea.

   b. _____ The chief complaint should be kept concise, with any additional information saved for the present illness history.

   c. _____ If possible, the chief complaint should be documented in the patient's own words.

   d. _____ The medical assistant should use accurate medical terminology when documenting the chief complaint.

   e. _____ The medical assistant may use diagnostic terminology when documenting the chief complaint.

   f. _____ The medical assistant should identify diseases when documenting the chief complaint.

   g. _____ It is important to obtain as complete a family history as possible to help with early diagnoses of familial diseases.

   h. _____ Familial diseases are those that affect blood relatives.

   i. _____ Documentation should be clear, concise, and correct.

   j. _____ It is acceptable to write over a mistake when you are documenting.

   k. _____ Any mistakes made during documentation should be dated and signed.

   l. _____ Documentation should occur immediately after a procedure is performed.

   m. _____ All documentation should be signed by the person who performed the task.

   n. _____ When you are documenting, it is acceptable to use abbreviations that are common in your local area, even if these are not commonly used in the medical office.

11. Subjective symptoms are sometimes simply called _____, whereas objective

    symptoms are called _____.

12. How are subjective symptoms obtained?

13. How are objective symptoms obtained?

14. Why is it important that the medical assistant ask questions of the patient in a private area rather than in the reception area?

Exercise 2

Online Activity—Obtaining a Medical History from a New Patient

30 minutes

* Sign in to Mountain View Clinic.
* From the patient list, select **Kevin McKinzie**.

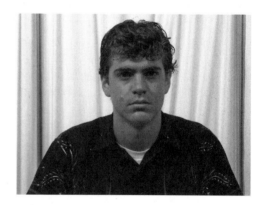

➡ • On the office map, click on **Reception**.

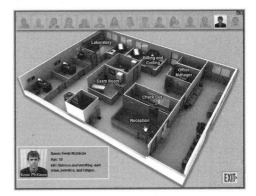

• Under the Watch heading, select **Patient Check-In** and view the video.

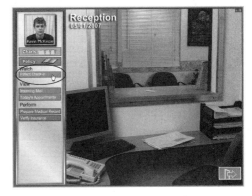

• Click **Close** at the end of the video to return to Reception.

1. Kevin McKinzie brings a history form to the medical office with him. What are the disadvantages of having the patient complete the medical history at home?

2. The administrative medical assistant takes the medical history and places it in a chart without reviewing it for completeness. Is this good practice? Explain your answer.

3. Would you have handled Mr. McKinzie's check-in differently? If yes, explain how. Did the medical assistant respond adequately to the patient's verbal and nonverbal communication?

- Click the exit arrow at the bottom right of the screen to leave the Reception area.
- On the Summary Menu, click **Return to Map**.
- On the office map, click on **Exam Room** to continue with Mr. McKinzie's visit.

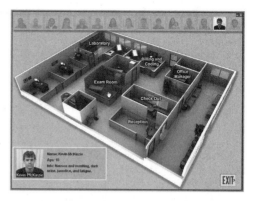

- From the menu on the left, click on **Charts** and select **1-General Health History Questionnaire** from the drop-down menu under the Patient Medical Information tab.

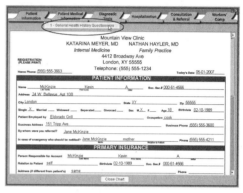

- Using the arrow at the top right of the questionnaire, turn to page 2.

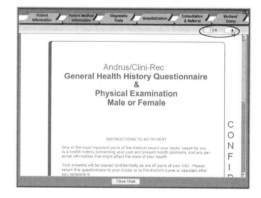

- Thoroughly review the information Mr. McKinzie provided on page 2 of the questionnaire.

4. What is the patient's chief complaint, as documented under Current Medical History?

5. What two areas of Mr. McKinzie's social history could have a bearing on this illness?

➤ • Again using the arrow at the top of the screen, turn to page 3 of the questionnaire.
   • Thoroughly review the information Kevin McKinzie provided regarding his past history.

   6. What, if any, familial history is relevant to his chief complaint?

➤ • Still in the chart, click on the **Patient
   Information** tab and select **1-Patient
   Information Form**.

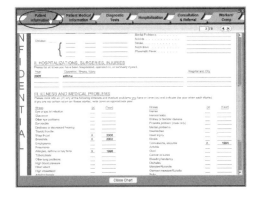

   • Read the Patient Information Form to find
     Mr. McKinzie's type of employment.
   • Click **Close Chart** to return to the Exam Room.
   • Click on **Exam Notes** (under View) and read the
     clinical diagnoses as documented by Dr. Hayler.

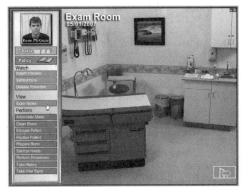

   • Click **Finish** to close the Exam Notes and return to the Exam Room.

   7. What are the indications for patient education and infection control for these clinical
      diagnoses?

- Click the exit arrow to leave the Exam Room.
- On the Summary Menu, click **Return to Map** and continue to the next exercise.

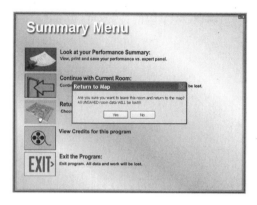

Exercise 3

Online Activity—Documentation of Chief Complaint for Established Patient

 30 minutes

- From the patient list, select **Hu Huang**. (*Note:* If you have exited the program, sign in again to Mountain View Clinic and select Hu Huang from the patient list.)

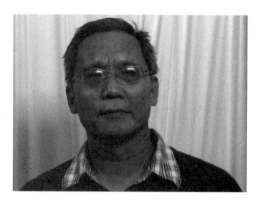

- On the office map, highlight and click on **Exam Room**.
- Under the Watch heading, select **Respiratory Care** to view the video.

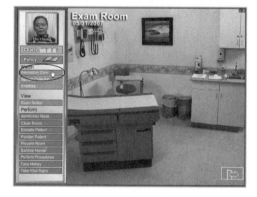

- Click **Close** at the end of the video to return to the Exam Room.
- Click on **Exam Notes** (under View) to read the documentation of Mr. Huang's visit.

1. What is your assessment of the verbal and nonverbal communication that Charlie displayed with Mr. Huang in the video?

2. What is the chief complaint for Mr. Huang?

3. Which of the symptoms listed are subjective symptoms?

4. What are the objective symptoms?

5. What other information could be placed in the History section of the Progress Notes?

6. Why was it important to obtain the information that Mr. Huang had been in China for several months?

- Click **Finish** to close the Exam Notes and return to the Exam Room.
- Click **Charts** to open Mr. Huang's medical record and select **1-Progress Notes** from the drop-down menu under the **Patient Medical Information** tab.

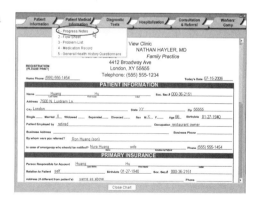

- Read the documentation from all of Mr. Huang's previous visits.

7. Based on your review of the Progress Notes for Mr. Huang's previous visits, what questions do you think would have been appropriate for the medical assistant to ask the patient regarding his medication compliance?

8. Indicate whether each of the following statements is true or false.

a. _____ The chief complaint for an established patient should be documented in Progress Notes unless a new history/physical exam form is being completed.

b. _____ When documenting the chief complaint in the medical record of an established patient, the same questions of when, where, how, and how long should be asked.

c. _____ After the physician identifies a diagnosis, it is permissible for the medical assistant to use that diagnosis in documentation of the chief complaint.

d. _____ Proper spelling is not as important when documenting the care of an established patient since the physician has already spelled the medical terminology correctly in earlier Progress Notes.

e. _____ Documentation for an established patient is just as important as for a new patient.

f. _____ If the medical office has unique guidelines concerning documentation, these are not as important as those you were taught in class and should not be followed.

g. _____ When documenting in any medical record, the extern or medical assisting student should sign the medical record with the designation of student medical assistant (SMA).

h. _____ The medical assistant should document both objective and subjective symptoms in the medical record.

i. _____ If the physician has used a local abbreviation in the medical record, it is acceptable for the medical assistant to also use this abbreviation, even if its use is not considered standard.

j. _____ Only clinical medical assistants document in medical records.

→ • Click **Close Chart** to return to the Exam Room.
   • Click the exit arrow to leave the Exam Room.
   • Select **Return to Map** from the Summary Menu.

Exercise 4

 Online Activity—Documentation by Administrative Medical Assistants

 15 minutes

- From the patient list, select **Tristan Tsosie**. (*Note:* If you have exited the program, sign in again to Mountain View Clinic and select Tristan Tsosie from the patient list.)

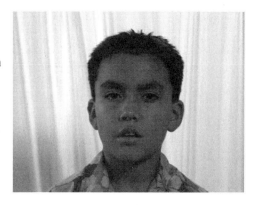

- On the office map, click on **Reception** to enter the check-in area.
- Under the Watch heading, click on **Patient Check-In** and view the video.

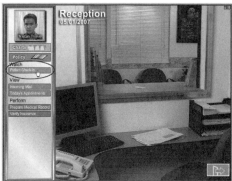

1. During the video, what important subjective symptoms does Tristan's sister report to the administrative medical assistant?

→ • Click the exit arrow to leave the Reception desk.
- Select **Return to Map** from the Summary Menu.
- Keeping Tristan as your patient, click on **Check Out** on the office map.

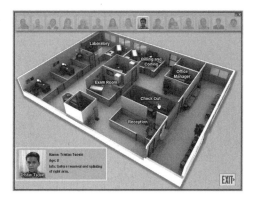

- Next, click **Charts** and select **1-Progress Notes** from under the **Patient Medical Information** tab.
- Read the initial documentation written by Dana Brick, CMA.

2. Which of the four questions that should be asked for accurate documentation of chief complaint has been omitted from the Progress Notes, even though Tristan's sister provided the needed information when Tristan was checked in?

3. Dana is a clinical medical assistant, and Kristin is an administrative medical assistant. Did the correct medical assistant document the information from the sister in the medical record?

4. What are your thoughts about the verbal and nonverbal communication that occurred among Kristin, Tristan, and Tristan's sister during check-in? Did Kristin communicate effectively? If you think there was a problem, how could it have been better handled?

- Click **Close Chart**; then click on the exit arrow.
- Select **Return to Map** from the Summary Menu and continue to the next exercise.

Exercise 5

 Writing Activity—Practicing Documentation of History and Chief Complaint

 45 minutes

- From the patient list, select **Wilson Metcalf**. (*Note:* If you have exited the program, sign in again to Mountain View Clinic and select Wilson Metcalf from the patient list.)

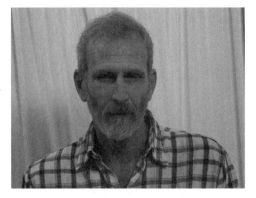

- On the office map, click on **Check Out**.
- Click on **Charts** and then select **1-Progress Notes** from the drop-down menu under the **Patient Medical Information** tab.
- Read the Progress Notes for Wilson Metcalf beginning with his initial visit to the office on 1/4/07.

1. According to the Progress Notes, what were Mr. Metcalf's drinking habits at the time of his visit on 1/4/07?

2. How much coffee did Mr. Metcalf admit to drinking in a day?

→ • Scroll down in the Progress Notes and read the documentation for the chief complaint for Mr. Metcalf's visit on 5/1/07.

3. What are Mr. Metcalf's drinking habits now?

4. How much coffee does he admit to drinking at this visit?

5. What was the diagnosis documented by Dr. Meyer on 1/4/07?

6. What is Mr. Metcalf's diagnosis on 5/1/07?

→ • Click on the **Patient Medical Information** tab again; this time, select **5-General Health History Questionnaire**.

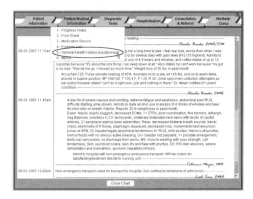

• Click on the arrow at the top right corner of the screen to turn to page 2.
• Read Wilson Metcalf's Health History form that was completed on 1/4/07.

7. Who do you think filled out the Health History form?

8. Under Section IV, General Health Attitude and Habits, what was Mr. Metcalf's response to the question about how much alcohol he drinks, if any?

9. According to the form, did Mr. Metcalf believe he had a problem with alcohol?

10. On this form, how much coffee does Mr. Metcalf say he drinks?

11. Are Wilson Metcalf's answers on the form consistent with the documentation in his Progress Notes? Explain. If the answers are not consistent, why do you think this may have happened?

12. Why would it have been important for the medical assistant to review this history with Wilson Metcalf?

13. Assume that you interviewed Wilson Metcalf on 1/4/07 and wrote the Progress Notes on that date. Complete the blank page of the General Health History Questionnaire below by answering the questions correctly for Mr. Metcalf based on the information he provided during the interview.

○   ○

ANDRUS/CLINI-REC   **HEALTH HISTORY QUESTIONNAIRE**

Chart No. _____

Identification Information   Today's Date _____

Name _____   Date of Birth _____

Occupation _____   Marital Status _____

PART A – PRESENT HEALTH HISTORY

I. CURRENT MEDICAL PROBLEMS

Please list the medical problems for which you came to see the doctor. About when did they begin?

Problems   Date Began
_____   _____
_____   _____
_____   _____

What concerns you most about these problems?
_____

If you are being treated for any other illness or medical problems by another physician, please describe the problems and write the name of the physician or medical facility treating you.

Illness or Medical Problem   Physician or Medical Facility   City
_____

II. MEDICATIONS

Please list all medications you are now taking, including those you buy without a doctor's prescription (such as aspirin, cold tablets or vitamin supplements).

_____   _____   _____
_____   _____   _____

III. ALLERGIES AND SENSITIVITIES

List anything that you are allergic to, such as certain foods, medications, dust, chemicals or soaps, household items, pollens, bee stings, etc., and indicate how each affects you.

Allergic To: Effect   Allergic To: Effect
_____   _____   _____   _____
_____   _____   _____   _____

IV. GENERAL HEALTH, ATTITUDE AND HABITS

How is your overall health now?	Health now: Poor ___ Fair ___ Good ___ Excellent ___
How has it been most of your life?	Health has been: Poor ___ Fair ___ Good ___ Excellent ___
In the past year:	
Has your appetite changed?	Appetite: Decreased ___ Increased ___ Stayed same ___
Has your weight changed?	Weight: Lost ___ lbs. Gained ___ lbs No change ___
Are you thirsty much of the time?	Thirsty: No ___ Yes ___
Has your "pep" changed?	Pep: Decreased ___ Increased ___ Stayed same ___
Do you usually have trouble sleeping?	Trouble sleeping: No ___ Yes ___
How much do you exercise?	Exercise: Little or none ___ Less than I need ___ All I need ___
Do you smoke?	Smokes: No ___ Yes ___ If yes, how many years? ___
How many each day?	___ Cigarettes ___ Cigars ___ Pipesfull
Have you ever smoked?	Smoked: No ___ Yes ___ If yes, how many years? ___
How many each day?	___ Cigarettes ___ Cigars ___ Pipesfull
Do you drink alchoholic beverages?	Alcohol: No ___ Yes ___ I drink ___ Beers ___ Glasses of wine ___ Drinks of hard liquor - day
Have you ever had a problem with alcohol?	Prior problem: No ___ Yes ___
How much coffee or tea do you usually drink?	Coffee/Tea: ___ cups of coffee or tea a day
Do you regularly wear seatbelts?	Seatbelts: No ___ Yes ___

DO YOU:	Rarely/Never	Occasionally	Frequently	DO YOU:	Rarely/Never	Occasionally	Frequently
Feel nervous?	___	___	___	Ever feel like commiting suicide?	___	___	___
Feel depressed?	___	___	___				
Find it hard to make decisions?	___	___	___	Feel bored with your life?	___	___	___
Lose your temper?	___	___	___	Use marijuana?	___	___	___
Worry a lot?	___	___	___	Use "hard drugs"?	___	___	___
Tire easily?	___	___	___	Do you want to talk to the doctor about a personal matter? No ___ Yes ___			
Have trouble relaxing?	___	___	___				
Have any sexual problems?	___	___	___				

C O N F I D E N T I A L

Created and Developed by "Medical Economics" Professional Systems
Copyright © 1979, 1983 Bibbero Systems International, Inc.   STOCK NO. 19-742-4   8/95   **Page 1**

14. Suppose that a patient named Mac Wallace (born 10/23/1980) comes to the office stating he has a fever and sore throat. He has had difficulty swallowing and has had pain in his right ear. All of these symptoms have lasted for about 4 days and have become progressively worse each day. He has also run out of blood pressure medicine and wants the prescription to be refilled. Before his throat became sore, his child had a case of strep throat. Document Mr. Wallace's chief complaint on the Progress Notes below.

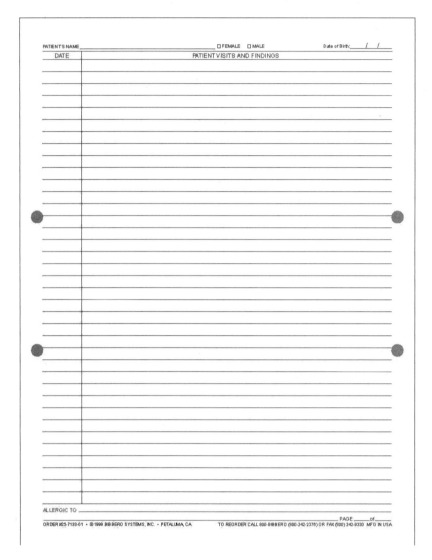

15. What subjective symptoms did Mr. Wallace report?

16. Which of these subjective symptoms could become objective symptoms following physical examination?

Patient Reception

👓 **Reading Assignment:** Chapter 37—Patient Reception

Patients: Teresa Hernandez, Wilson Metcalf

Learning Objectives:

- Discuss measures to protect the confidentiality of patients in the reception area.
- List information that must be obtained from new patients.
- Describe the proper check-in procedures for new and established patients.
- Discuss procedures necessary to verify whether a patient's insurance will pay for services.

Overview:

In this lesson you will observe Kristin, the medical assistant, as she performs reception duties and assists with registering a new patient and an established patient. Verification of patient insurance information and completion of required paperwork are covered. You will view the check-out procedure with patient Teresa Hernandez and observe how the copay is collected and how her next visit is scheduled. Also addressed is the importance of confidentiality while registering patients to ensure that their privacy is protected.

Exercise 1

Online Activity—Maintaining Confidentiality

30 minutes

- Sign in to Mountain View Clinic.
- Select **Teresa Hernandez** from the patient list. (*Note:* If you have exited the program, sign in again to Mountain View Clinic and select Teresa Hernandez from the patient list.)

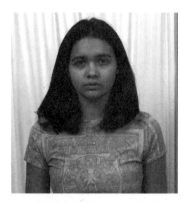

- On the office map, click on **Reception**.

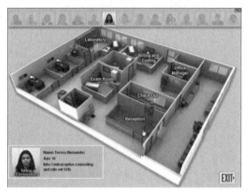

- Under the Watch heading, select **Patient Check-In** to view the video.

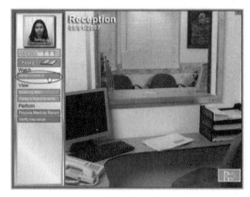

- At the end of the video, click **Close** to return to the Reception desk.

1. As Teresa was checking in, did Kristin take all the necessary steps to protect Teresa's confidential health information? Explain.

2. What additional steps could Kristin have taken to ensure Teresa's privacy was protected?

3. What form was Kristin referring to in the video, and what is the purpose of this form?

4. According to Teresa, she is covered by her father's insurance. Can she request that the insurance company send the Explanation of Benefits (EOB) for her visit to an address other than the guarantor's? Why or why not?

➤ • Remain in the Reception area with Teresa Hernandez as your patient and continue to the next exercise.

Exercise 2

 Online Activity—Check-In Procedure for a New Patient

 15 minutes

- In the Reception area, click on the **Computer** to view Today's Appointments and review the schedule.

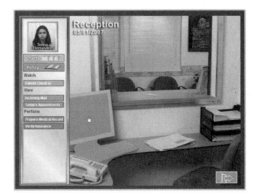

- Scroll down the page to locate Teresa Hernandez's name on the schedule.

1. What time is Teresa's scheduled appointment?

2. There is a notation next to Teresa's name in the appointment book. What is the notation, and what does it mean?

→ - Click **Finish** to close the Appointment Book and return to the Reception desk.
- Now click on the **Insurance Card** (lying on the counter of the Reception window); this activates the **Verify Insurance** wizard.
- Select the appropriate question to ask Teresa.
- Identify the correct steps in the insurance verification process for the patient by clicking in the appropriate boxes.
- At the bottom of this screen, under View, click **Insurance Card(s)** to see the back and front of Teresa's insurance card.
- Make a notation of the copayment amount for the visit, which is listed on the front of the card (next to PCP).
- Click **Finish** to return to the Reception desk.

3. What information does Kristin need to get from Teresa based on her response about her insurance coverage?

4. If Mountain View Clinic is using electronic patient records, how would Kristin input a copy of the insurance card information into the electronic system.

5. What other information should Kristin request?

6. Why is this necessary?

→ • Click the exit arrow to leave the Reception area. On the Summary Menu, click **Return to Map**. Keeping Teresa Hernandez as your patient, click to enter the **Check Out** area.
• Under the Watch heading, select **Patient Check-Out** to view the video.

7. How much is Teresa's copayment amount for today's visit?

8. How did the medical assistant know this?

9. What other task did the medical assistant perform before Teresa left the office?

→ • Click the exit arrow and select **Return to Map**.

Exercise 3

Online Activity—Performing Check-In Procedures for an Established Patient

20 minutes

- From the patient list, select **Wilson Metcalf**. (*Note:* If you have exited the program, sign in again to Mountain View Clinic and select Wilson Metcalf from the patient list.)

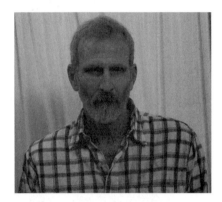

- On the office map, click on **Reception**.
- Under Watch, select **Patient Check-In** to view the check-in video.
- When Kristin closes the window on Mr. Metcalf, stop the video and click **Close**.

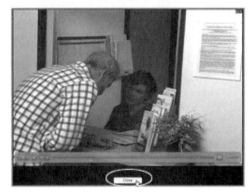

- At the Reception desk, click on the **Insurance Card** on the window counter to perform the Verify Insurance task.
- Ask the appropriate question of Mr. Metcalf.
- Leave the Verify Insurance window open as you complete the following questions.

1. Mr. Metcalf has two insurance cards. Why should the Medicare card be the one filed for this visit?

2. What information does Kristin need to obtain from Mr. Metcalf based on his response?

3. Using the blank Primary Insurance section of the Patient Information Form below, update Mr. Metcalf's insurance information. (*Note:* The new insurance cards can be viewed in the Verify Insurance window.)

PRIMARY INSURANCE

Person Responsible for Account _____
                                    Last Name   First Name   Initial

Relation to Patient _____ Birthdate _____ Soc. Sec.# _____

Address (if different from patient's) _____ Phone _____

City _____ State _____ Zip _____

Person Responsible Employed by _____ Occupation _____

Business Address _____ Business Phone _____

Insurance Company _____

Contract # _____ Group # _____ Subscriber # _____

Name of other dependents covered under this plan _____

ADDITIONAL INSURANCE

Is patient covered by additional insurance? _____ Yes _____ No

Subscriber Name _____ Relation to Patient _____ Birthdate _____

Address (if different from patient's) _____ Phone _____

City _____ State _____ Zip _____

Subscriber Employed by _____ Business Phone _____

Insurance Company _____ Soc. Sec.# _____

Contract # _____ Group # _____ Subscriber # _____

Name of other dependents covered under this plan

View:

> Insurance Card(s)
>
> Patient Information Form
>
> Computer Information

<< Back   Finish

Scheduling and Managing Appointments

Reading Assignment: Chapter 40—Scheduling Appointments

Patient: Janet Jones

Learning Objectives:

- Discuss the rationale for providing space in a day's appointment schedule for emergency appointments.
- Explain the need for a matrix on the appointment schedule.
- Describe the role of the Policy Manual in appointment scheduling.
- Explain the importance of verbal communication concerning appointment delays.
- Apply the skills of scheduling appointments in person and by telephone.
- Apply the skills of maintaining the appointment book.
- Identify office policies concerning rescheduling appointments.
- Apply the skills of rescheduling appointments.

Overview:

In this lesson you will schedule and manage appointments using the policies established for this office. The patient, Janet Jones, is upset because she has not been seen immediately. You will discuss the proper way to deal with such a situation. After today's appointment, Janet Jones will need to come back for a follow-up appointment. You will schedule this appointment for her at the appropriate time and schedule other appointments for established and new patients.

Exercise 1

Online Activity—Using a Specific Daily Appointment Schedule

20 minutes

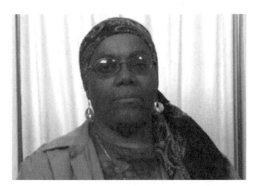

- Sign in to Mountain View Clinic
- From the patient list, select **Janet Jones**.

- On the office map, click on **Reception**.
- At the Reception desk, click the **Computer** to open the appointment book. (*Note:* You can also do this by clicking on **Today's Appointments** under View on the Room Menu.) Review the schedule, noting the time of Janet Jones' appointment. You will need to scroll down the appointment book to see the entire day.

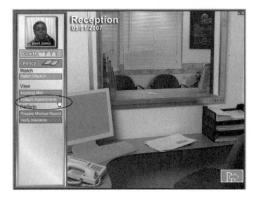

- Click **Finish** to close the appointment book and return to the Reception desk.

1. According to the appointment schedule, what time is Janet Jones' appointment?

2. If Janet Jones signed in at 1:30 p.m., would she have been on time for her appointment? Explain your answer.

• Under the Watch heading, click **Patient Check-In** and watch the video.
  • Click **Close** at the end of the video to return to the Reception desk.

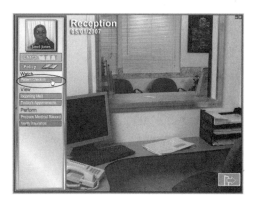

3. Janet Jones is upset when she arrives at the counter. How does Kristin handle the patient in a professional way through verbal and nonverbal communication?

4. Assuming that Ms. Jones checked in at 1:30 p.m., what would have been an appropriate statement for the receptionist to make to the patient as she checked in to prevent her from becoming so upset?

  • At the Reception desk, click on **Policy** to open the office Policy Manual.

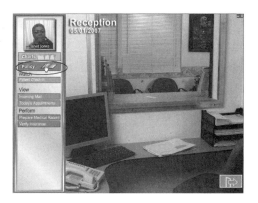

→ • Type "appointment scheduling" in the search bar and click on the magnifying glass.

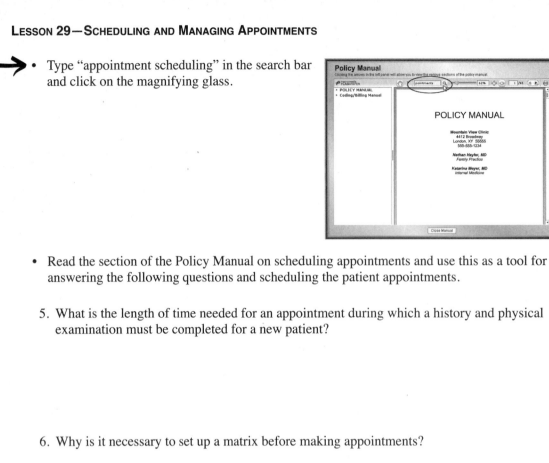

• Read the section of the Policy Manual on scheduling appointments and use this as a tool for answering the following questions and scheduling the patient appointments.

5. What is the length of time needed for an appointment during which a history and physical examination must be completed for a new patient?

6. Why is it necessary to set up a matrix before making appointments?

7. What buffer times are available for emergency appointments?

8. According to the office Policy Manual, what would have been appropriate concerning rescheduling Janet Jones' appointment?

9. Why is it important to identify workers' compensation appointments at the time of scheduling rather than at the time of the appointment?

10. Is the patient's time just as valuable as the physician's time?

- Click **Close Manual** to return to the Reception desk.
- Leave the Reception area by clicking the exit arrow at the lower right corner of the screen.

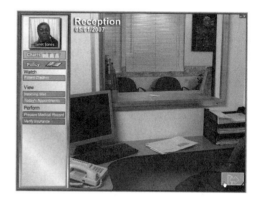

- At the Summary Menu, select **Return to Map** and continue to the next exercise.

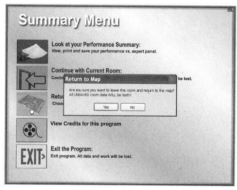

Exercise 2

 Writing Activity—Adding Appointments to a Schedule

20 minutes

At the end of the day on April 31, a list of patients needing appointments on May 1 was shown to Dr. Hayler and Dr. Meyer. Both physicians stated that because few patients were currently in the hospital, they would be able to see patients in the clinic earlier than usual the next morning. Dr. Hayler and Dr. Meyer will begin seeing patients at 8:15 a.m. The staff has been informed of the early start. Your job is to add the appointments to the schedule. The white areas of the appointment book indicate buffer times for adding patients who need to see the doctor today or for those patients with emergent needs. To determine how much time you need to block off for appointments, select a patient from the patient list, go to the Reception desk, open the Policy Manual, and type "appointment scheduling" in the search bar to review the office policy for allotting appointment times.

1. a. Insert the following appointments for Dr. Hayler onto the morning schedule on the next page.

 (1) Robert Leuker is a patient who has not been to the clinic in 5 years and wants to be seen for a lump in his arm. He has a past history of cancer and needs to be seen ASAP. He should be seen first in the morning so that he can be referred as necessary. He is insured through BlueCross/BlueShield (BC/BS). His phone number is (555) 555-8890.

 (2) Lindsey Repp needs a follow-up appointment for an earache and recurrent fever. She is insured through Central Health HMO and can be double-booked at the end of the appointment for Louise Parlet. Her telephone number is (555) 555-9004.

 (3) John Price, who needs a follow-up appointment for his blood pressure, has Medicare. His blood pressure was low when he took it yesterday, and he feels dizzy. He simply wants Dr. Hayler to reevaluate his medication. He can be seen just before lunch. Mr. Price's phone number is (555) 555-1998.

5/1/20XX	Dr. Hayler			Dr. Meyer	
Time	Patient Name	Insurance		Patient Name	Insurance
8:00 AM	(Hospital rounds) Joe Smitty - Chem 12, CBC Marsha Brady - Fasting BS			(Hospital Rounds)	
8:15 AM	(Hospital rounds)			(Hospital Rounds) Joanne Crosby, PT, PTT	
8:30 AM	Louise Parlet, Est. Pt New Pregnancy/Pelvic (555) 555-3214	Teachers		Rhea Davison, Est. Pt. Elevated BS, abdominal distention, pelvic (555) 555-5656	None
8:45 AM					
9:00 AM					
9:15 AM					
9:30 AM				Hu Huang, Est. Pt. Severe cough, fever (555) 555-1454	Medicare
9:45 AM	Jade Wong, NP 7 mos well child checkup/ immunization (555) 555-3345	Central Health HMO			
10:00 AM				~~Chris O'Neill - back pain~~ (pt cancelled - resched 5/7) Jesus Santo, Walk-in Leg pain, SOB	None
10:15 AM					
10:30 AM				Jean Deere, Est. Pt. Memory loss, ear pain (555) 555-6361	Medicare
10:45 AM	Tristan Tsosie, Est. Pt. Suture Removal (555) 555-1515	Blue Cross/ Blue Shield			
11:00 AM					
11:15 AM				Wilson Metcalf, Est. Pt. N/V, abdominal pain, difficulty urinating - (555) 555-3311	Medicare
11:30 AM	LUNCH				
11:45 AM					
12:00 PM					
12:15 PM	Renee Anderson, NP Annual GYN Exam (555) 555-3331	Blue Cross/ Blue Shield			

b. After completing Dr. Hayler's appointments, add the following appointments for Dr. Meyer in the morning, using the same schedule on the previous page.

(1) Catherine Lake needs a follow-up appointment for pyelonephritis. She forgot to make this follow-up appointment when she was last seen. Ms. Lake is going out of town for 2 weeks and needs to see Dr. Meyer before leaving. Her insurance coverage is through BC/BS. Dr. Meyer will see her at the earliest appointment time. Catherine Lake's phone number is (555) 555-1865.

(2) Lucille Meryl needs to be seen for a follow-up to a thyroid test. Dr. Meyer wants to see her as a double-booking at the end of the appointment for Rhea Davison. Her insurance is through Drake. Her phone number is (555) 555-3219.

(3) An established patient, Simon Reed, calls at 11:30 a.m. to tell you that he has some chest pain, and even though he has an appointment for tomorrow, he does not think he should wait. Mr. Reed has experienced a heart attack in the past. When you discuss this with Dr. Meyer, she tells you to phone 911 while keeping the patient on the line. She also says that she will go to the hospital to see Mr. Reed once he has arrived at the emergency department. What notation should you make on the schedule?

2. You must now call John Price to inform him that Dr. Hayler will see him just before lunch. What information will need to be given to Mr. Price. Why did Dr. Hayler need to be contacted before making the appointment for Mr. Price?

3. You must also call Lucille Meryl to inform her that Dr. Meyer wants to see her about her test results. What information do you need to provide? What will you say to her if she asks why she needs to be seen so quickly?

Exercise 3

Online Activity—Preparing an Appointment Schedule

30 minutes

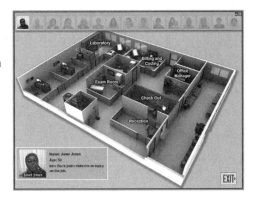

- In this exercise you will continue with Janet Jones' visit. If you are already at the office map, click on **Check Out** to go to the Check Out desk. (*Note:* If you have exited the program, sign in again to Mountain View Clinic, select Janet Jones, and go to the Check Out desk.)

- At the Check Out desk, click on the **Encounter Form** (the clipboard on the desk). Scroll down the document to review the entire form.

1. What is the date that Janet Jones should return to the clinic for a follow-up appointment?

2. How much time should be allotted to the follow-up appointment for Ms. Jones?

3. For what time of the day was Ms. Jones' follow-up appointment scheduled?

Your next job is to prepare the appointment schedule for the day. Use the blank pages of the appointment book in questions 4 and 5 on the next two pages to complete the following activities:

(1) Set up the appointment sheet for the date that Janet Jones is to return for her follow-up visit, using the same time the medical assistant in the video scheduled this appointment.

(2) Using the information in the Policy Manual, set up the matrix for that day. (*Note:* If you need to review this, return to the Policy Manual, type "hours of operation" in the search bar, and click on the magnifying glass.)

(3) Add an appointment at 11:00 a.m. for Kay Soto (an established patient) with Dr. Meyer. Ms. Soto has been prescribed a weight loss program and is coming in for a weight check. Her insurance is through Metro HMO. Ms. Soto's phone number is (555) 555-0054.

This list of tasks continues at the top of page 328. Go to that page and continuing adding appointments or making adjustments to the schedule as instructed.

4.

Appointment Book, Page 1

/ /20XX	Dr. Hayler		Dr. Meyer	
Time	Patient Name	Insurance	Patient Name	Insurance
8:00 AM				
8:15 AM				
8:30 AM				
8:45 AM				
9:00 AM				
9:15 AM				
9:30 AM				
9:45 AM				
10:00 AM				
10:15 AM				
10:30 AM				
10:45 AM				
11:00 AM				
11:15 AM				
11:30 AM				
11:45 AM				
12:00 PM				
12:15 PM				

5.

Appointment Book, Page 2

/ /20XX	Dr. Hayler		Dr. Meyer	
Time	Patient Name	Insurance	Patient Name	Insurance
12:30 PM				
12:45 PM				
1:00 PM				
1:15 PM				
1:30 PM				
1:45 PM				
2:00 PM				
2:15 PM				
2:30 PM				
2:45 PM				
3:00 PM				
3:15 PM				
3:30 PM				
3:45 PM				
4:00 PM				
4:15 PM				
4:30 PM				
4:45 PM				
5:00 PM				

Continue your scheduling by adding the following appointments or adjustments to the forms on the previous two pages.

(4) George Smith, age 15, is to be seen by Dr. Hayler for a football injury he incurred the night before. He has State Agricultural Insurance and is an existing patient. George needs to be seen as early as possible so that he can go to school. Mr. Smith's phone number is (555) 555-8778.

(5) Callie Agree, a new patient, is to be seen for a possible sinus infection. She has Medicare and will be accompanied by her daughter. The daughter prefers to see Dr. Meyer in the midmorning so that her mother will have adequate time to dress. Ms. Agree's phone number is (555) 555-3452.

(6) Sophie Coats, age 6 months, is an established patient who will be seen by Dr. Hayler for a well-baby visit. She is due to have immunizations at this visit. Schedule Sophie for a 60-minute appointment. Her mother prefers to have an appointment as early in the morning as possible. Sophie is covered by her father's insurance through Banker's Health. Ms. Coats' phone number is (555) 554-0090.

(7) Mamie Mack, age 18, is an established patient who needs a physical examination for college. She prefers to be seen by Dr. Hayler. Either late morning or early afternoon is better for her since she is still in school. She is covered through George Allen Insurance at her mother's place of employment. Ms. Mack's phone number is (555) 554-8745.

(8) Kay Soto calls to cancel her appointment for the day because she has to leave town to take care of her ill mother. She does not want to reschedule at this time.

(9) Dr. Hayler will need to leave at 11:15 a.m. for a dental appointment but will be back in the afternoon. Mark this on the appointment sheet.

(10) Dr. Meyer is scheduled to be off the afternoon of this day. Mark this on the appointment sheet.

6. What is the necessary procedure for canceling Kay Soto's appointment?
   a. Erase the canceled appointment and tell Ms. Soto that there will be a charge because she did not give 24 hours' notice.
   b. Cross out the appointment (using the office-preferred writing implement) and record the cancellation in the patient medical record.
   c. Report the cancellation to Dr. Meyer.
   d. Tell her that she must reschedule this appointment today if she wants to continue her medical care at the clinic.

7. Why is it important to document a canceled appointment in the patient's medical record?

Filing Medical Records

/OℛD **Reading Assignment:** Chapter 41—Medical Records Management

Patients: All

Learning Objectives:

- Alphabetize patient names for efficiency in filing medical records.
- List the necessary steps needed to prepare a paper medical record for filing.
- Describe the use of color coding to enhance paper medical record systems.
- Identify the filing systems used most frequently in the medical office for patient records.
- Discuss the differences between alphabetic and numeric filing systems.
- Determine which patients are established patients and which are new patients for the purpose of preparing charts.
- Discuss the methods for finding displaced paper medical records.
- Explain the most important features of an electronic medical record (EMR) system.

Overview:

Proper filing of medical records is essential in providing continuity of care for patients. In this lesson you will determine whether patients are new or established in preparation for filing. You will be asked to differentiate between alphabetic and numeric filing systems and identify methods for locating misplaced medical information. Also discussed are the most important features of a typical EMR system.

329

Exercise 1

Online Activity—Preparing Patient Medical Records for Filing

50 minutes

- Sign in to Mountain View Clinic.
- One at a time, click on each patient's photograph on the patient list (moving from left to right) and record the patient's name in the table in question 1 below.

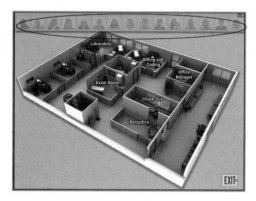

1. Record the names of all the Mountain View Clinic patients in the first and third columns of the table below. (*Note:* Fill in all of column 1 first; then continue at the top of column 3. You will complete the remaining columns later.)

Patient Name; NP or Est. Pt.	First Date of Service; Last Date of Service	Patient Name; NP or Est. Pt.	First Date of Service; Last Date of Service

• Now click again on any patient in the patient list. Then on the office map, click on **Reception**. At the Reception desk, click on the **Computer** to open the Today's Appointments window. Find a patient's name and then, next to this patient's name in the table in question 1, indicate whether that patient is a new patient (write *NP*) or an established patient (write *Est. Pt.*) (*Note:* You will fill in the columns 2 and 4 later.)

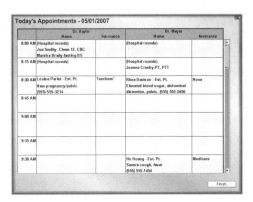

2. With the Today's Appointments window still open, make a list below of the patients Dr. Hayler is to see in the morning. List these patients in the correct order for their appointments and note whether the medical record can be pulled from the files of established patients or whether a new record should be prepared.

3. What medical records will need to be pulled from the files for Dr. Meyer's morning patients? Will any of these patients need to have a new record prepared? List these patients and their record needs below (in the order of their appointment times).

• Click **Finish** to close the appointment book and return to the Reception desk.
• Click the exit arrow in right lower corner of screen.

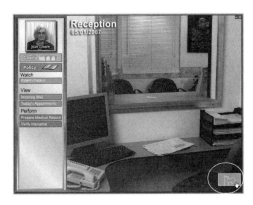

• From the Summary Menu, click on **Return to Map**; then click **Yes** to return to the office map and select another patient.

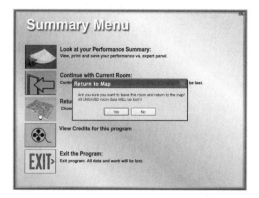

• Beginning with the first patient on the left in the patient list, click on **Reception**. Open the patient's chart, click on the **Patient Medical Information** tab, and select **1-Progress Notes**. Based on what you find, record the patient's first and last dates of service in the table in question 1 (column 2 or 4, depending on the patient).

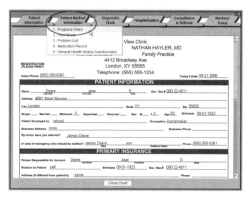

• *Important:* New patients will not have any forms in their chart. Use today's virtual date— 5/1/07—as their first date of service; there will be no "last date of service" for new patients.

• When you have recorded the date(s) for the first patient, click **Close Chart**; then click the exit arrow. From the Summary Menu, click on **Return to Map**.

• Select your next patient, open the chart, and record the date(s) in the table.

• Continue these steps for each patient until you have completed the table in question 1.

4. Using the table in question 1 as a reference, list the patients' names in alphabetic order in the left column below. In the right column indicate whether the medical records for each patient will be available in the file cabinet of established patients or whether the record will need to be organized and placed in the correct position as a new medical record.

Alphabetic List of Patients   **New or Established Record?**

5. As you pull the medical records for established patients, you will need to change the year on their medical records (unless the patient has already been seen in the current year). List the established patients below and indicate what year will need to be relabeled on their medical record (if this applies).

Name of Established Patient	Year That Will Need to Be Relabeled

6. At the end of the morning, the medical records need to be filed correctly to prevent loss and to ensure proper time management. Below, list in alphabetic order the names of patients who had morning appointments today and whose records will need to be refiled.

Exercise 2

Writing Activity

25 minutes

Answer the following questions regarding paper medical records and electronic medical record (EMR) systems.

1. Which supply would not be used to help prevent misfiling of paper medical records?
   a. Colored letter tabs for use with names
   b. Colored tabs for the last year seen in the office
   c. Outguides
   d. Alphabet tabs in the filing system

2. The two filing systems most often used in a medical office are _____ and

   _____ filing.

3. Describe the differences between alphabetic and numeric filing systems.

4. How are EMR systems updated with patient information?

5. When paper records are scanned into an EMR system, what should the medical assistant do with the paper record?

Written Communication

Reading Assignment: Chapter 42—Written Communications
Chapter 43—Mail

Patient: Wilson Metcalf

Learning Objectives:

- Prepare letters in response to the mail received.
- Use correct grammar, spelling, and formatting techniques in letter writing.
- Read mail correspondence correctly.

Overview:

This lesson discusses the importance of clear, written communication. You will practice writing correspondence that is grammatically correct and that provides an appropriate response to vendors and patients.

Exercise 1

Online Activity—Composing a Letter for an NSF Check

40 minutes

- Sign in to Mountain View Clinic.
- From the patient list, select **Wilson Metcalf**.

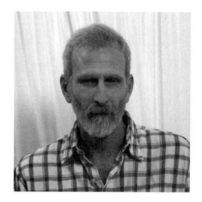

- On the office map, highlight and click on **Reception** to enter the Reception area.

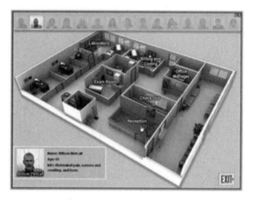

- Click the **Stackable Trays** to view the mail received by the clinic.
- Click the numbers to examine and read each piece of mail.

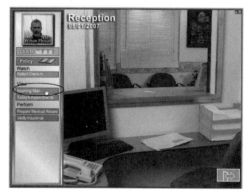

1. Were any payments received in the mail today?

2. List the people from whom payments were received.

3. What is the name of the physician who sent a consultation letter to Dr. Meyer?

4. The consultation letter was written in reference to what patient?

→ • From the list of mail at the top of the screen, click on **7** to view that piece of mail again.

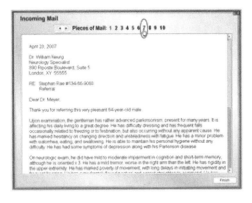

5. Below, write your letter to the patient about the NSF check, using an acceptable format. Be sure your message conveys the need to handle this matter within a certain number of days. Also make it clear that no further checks will be accepted for this patient's medical care at Mountain View Clinic. This letter should be prepared for a signature by the office manager.

Mountain View Clinic

4412 Broadway / London, XY 55555 / Phone: (555) 555-1234 / Fax: (555) 555-1239

Nathan Hayler, MD - Family Practice / Katarina Meyer, MD - Internal Medicine

→ • Keep the Incoming Mail window open and continue to the next exercise.

Exercise 2

Online Activity—Composing a Letter in Response to an Inaccurate Accounts Payable Notice

 15 minutes

- From the list of mail at the top of the screen, click on **10** to read the letter from Summer Oxygen Company.
- Click **Finish** to return to the Reception Desk.

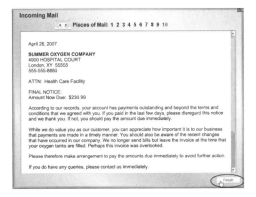

- Click the exit arrow to leave the Reception area.
- On the Summary Menu, click **Return to Map**.

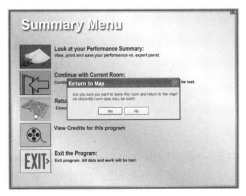

- On the office map, highlight and click on **Office Manager** to enter the manager's office.

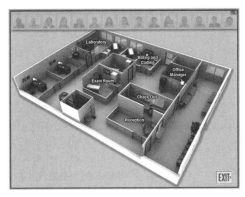

- Click on the **Bank Statement** (green file folder on the desk) to view the Clinic's most recent statement from the bank.

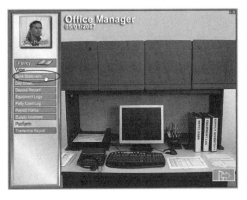

• In the Bank Statement window, select the **Check Ledger** tab to review the most recent checks written by Mountain View Clinic.

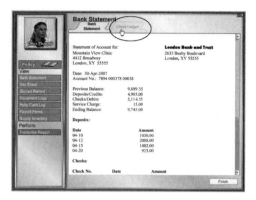

1. There was a payment made to Summer Oxygen Company for $230.99.

   a. According to the check ledger, what was the date this payment was made?

   b. What was the check number?

• Click on the **Bank Statement** tab to review the account activity for April 2007. Scroll down to see the entire statement.

2. Did check #1230 for $230.99 clear the account, according to the bank statement?

• While the Bank Statement window is open, compose a rough draft for a letter to the oxygen supply company in response to the claim that the invoice has not been paid. Be sure to include in the correspondence that a copy of the canceled check is enclosed with the letter.

• Click **Finish** to return to the Office Manager area.

3. Below, write your letter to the oxygen company using an acceptable format. Be sure your message includes all information needed to clear the accounts payable. This letter should be prepared for signature by the office manager.

Mountain View Clinic

4412 Broadway / London, XY 55555 / Phone: (555) 555-1234 / Fax (555) 555-1239

Nathan Hayler, MD - Family Practice / Katarina Meyer, MD - Internal Medicine

Exercise 3

Online Activity—Writing a Termination Letter

30 minutes

- Sign in to Mountain View Clinic.
- Select **Wilson Metcalf** from the patient list. (*Note:* You will not interact with Mr. Metcalf or any other patient during this exercise, but in order to access the office schedule in the Reception area, a patient must be selected.)
- From the office map, click on **Reception**.
- At the Reception desk, click on the **Computer** to review the day's schedule. You will need to scroll down the appointment book to see both the morning and afternoon schedules.

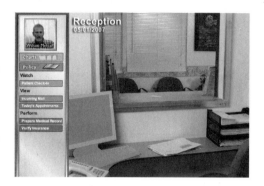

1. What is the name of the patient who has canceled an appointment, and what was the patient's chief complaint?

Use the following steps to find Mountain View Clinic's policy regarding canceled appointments.

 • Click **Finish** to close the appointment book and return to the Reception desk. Click on **Policy** to open the office Policy Manual.

- Type "cancel" in the search bar and click the magnifying glass to read the office policy regarding canceled appointments.
- Click **Close Manual** to return to the Reception desk.

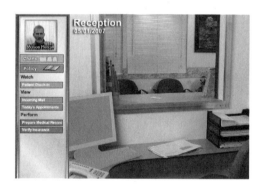

2. What is the role of the medical assistant in providing information about cancellations to the physician?

3. According to the Policy Manual, what is the next step to be taken with this patient, who has canceled his last three appointments? Explain your answer.

4. Below, compose a letter to the patient you identified in question 1. In the letter, describe the reason for possible termination and the necessary steps needed to remain a patient of Dr. Meyer. The letter should include all of the reasons for possible termination and the need for the patient to keep appointments as scheduled. The letter can also state that Dr. Meyer is concerned about continuity of care and its importance to the safety of all patients.

Mountain View Clinic

4412 Broadway / London, XY 55555 / Phone: (555) 555-1234 / Fax: (555) 555-1239

Nathan Hayler, MD - Family Practice / Katarina Meyer, MD - Internal Medicine

Critical Thinking Question

5. Why does the letter you composed in question 4 need to be sent by certified mail?

Critical Thinking Question

6. If a decision is made to terminate a patient, how much time must be allowed between notification and the termination?

Bookkeeping

Reading Assignment: Chapter 44—Managing Practice Finances
Chapter 47—Billing and Collection

Patients: All

Learning Objectives:

- Post daily entries on the day sheet and prepare bank deposits at the end of the day.
- Process credit balances, NSF checks, and checks from collection agencies.
- Process credit balances and complete necessary steps to process a refund, including preparation of a check.
- Reconcile a bank statement.
- Maintain a petty cash fund.
- Discuss the maintenance of records for accounting and banking purposes.
- Discuss the importance of managing accounts payable promptly.

Overview:

In this lesson you will perform all the basic bookkeeping procedures for the office. All patients will be added to the day sheet, along with the payments and the NSF check received in today's mail. A deposit record will be prepared. The steps for reconciliation of the bank statement and maintenance of records for accounting purposes will also be covered.

Exercise 1

Online Activity—Posting Charges to Ledger Cards

30 minutes

- Sign in to Mountain View Clinic.
- Select **Jade Wong** from the patient list.

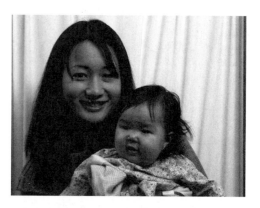

- On the office map, highlight and click on **Billing and Coding**.
- In the Billing and Coding office, select the **Encounter Form** on the desk to review the services that will be billed for Jade's visit.

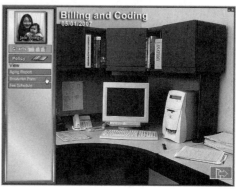

1. a. Using the Encounter Form for Jade Wong, begin completing the blank ledger card below.
   b. In the column marked Professional Service, list each individual service provided, but do not enter any fee or balance information.
   c. After the last service has been entered, be sure to document that the copay was collected and enter the copay amount in the Payment column.

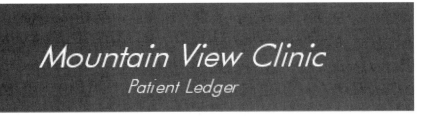

Patient Name:

Insurance Type:

Date	Professional Service	Fee ($)	Payment ($)	Adj. ($)	Prev. Bal. ($)	New Balance ($)
Totals						

• Click **Finish** to return to Billing and Coding.

• Now click on the **Fee Schedule** (hanging on the wall) to review the fees that Mountain View Clinic charges for various services and procedures.

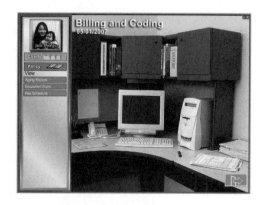

• Using the ledger card form in question 1, fill in the fees charged for the listed services; then calculate the balances. (*Note:* The balance should be adjusted line by line as each service or payment is added or subtracted.)

2. After filling in the services, charges, and payments for Jade's current visit, should the ledger card be totaled as indicated at the bottom of the card? Explain your answer.

• Click **Finish** to close the Fee Schedule; then click the exit arrow to leave Billing and Coding.

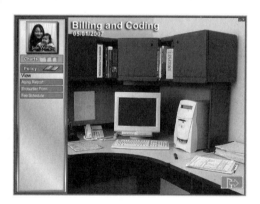

• On the Summary Menu, click on **Return to Map** and continue to the next exercise.

Exercise 2

 Online Activity—Posting Entries to a Day Sheet

 60 minutes

1. In this activity you will post charges and payments for the patients who were seen in the office today, using the blank day sheet provided on the next page. Note that the Distribution column indicates which physician, Dr. Hayler or Dr. Meyer, provided care to the patient. The amount of money the patient paid should be recorded in one of those columns, in addition to the Payment column.

   a. In the Patient Name column on the blank day sheet, list the patients in the following order: Jade Wong, Louise Parlet, Hu Huang, Rhea Davison, Jesus Santo, Jean Deere, Tristan Tsosie, Wilson Metcalf, Renee Anderson, Jose Imero, Shaunti Begay, Janet Jones, Kevin McKinzie, John R. Simmons, and Teresa Hernandez.

   b. The first patient listed on your day sheet is Jade Wong. Select **Jade Wong** from the patient list. Then click on **Check Out** on the office map. Once in the Check Out area, click on the **Encounter Form** clipboard.

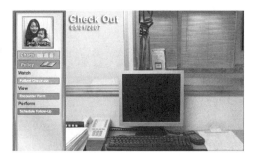

   c. Complete each column for Jade Wong on the day sheet using the Total Charges, Previous Balance, and Amount Received information listed on her Encounter Form. Refer back to the ledger card in Exercise 1 to confirm your totals. (*Note:* Unlike the ledger card, the Professional Service column on the day sheet is a summary description of the visit.)

   d. Also, make a note next to the patient's name to indicate whether the patient paid by cash, check, or credit card. If payment was made by check, include the check number.

   e. Repeat the previous steps for each patient (i.e., select the patient, go to Check Out, open the Encounter Form, fill in the Day Sheet). As you finish each patient's portion of the day sheet, click Finish to close the Encounter Form. Click the exit arrow to leave Check Out and Return to Map to select the next patient.

   f. When you have finished recording the information for the last patient on the list, return to the office map.

Mountain View Clinic
Daysheet

Date	Professional Service	Fee	Payment	Adjustment	New Balance	Old Balance	Patient's Name	Distribution Dr. Hayler	Dr. Meyer

TOTALS

• From the office map, click on **Reception**. (*Note:* The selected patient should be Teresa Hernandez, the last patient on your list in question 1.)

• At the Reception desk, click on the **Stackable Trays** to open the Incoming Mail window and to view the day's correspondence.

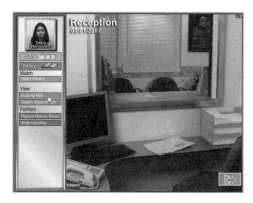

2. a. View each piece of incoming mail; then on the blank day sheet below, record any patient payments received by the clinic and any charges paid by the clinic in the appropriate columns.

   b. Be sure to include a description of the payment/charge and the patient's name.

   c. For any check payments, make a note of the bank and check number next to the patient's name.

   d. To complete the remaining columns, first click **Finish** to close the mail.

   e. Next, click the exit arrow and select **Return to Map**.

   f. Click on **Office Manager** and then on the **Day Sheet** on the desk (to the right of the computer keyboard) to find any previous balance information. Then recalculate the balance and record in the New Balance column.

   g. Mark Bonsel's previous account balance was zero ("0") before you received the NSF check. The NSF check shows that it was paid on April 7, 2007, but it does not indicate what it was for, other than a balance. Assume it was for a level II new patient visit, which would be $65.00 on the date of April 7, 2007. (*Note:* A copy of Sarah Anita's EOB from Blue Cross/Blue Shield was also received in the mail. The insurance payment and adjustment related to this EOB have already been posted on the day sheet and ledger card in the office manager's area. Thus this piece of mail will not need to be posted again.)

   h. Recalculate the balance and record it in the New Balance column.

Mountain View Clinic
Daysheet

Date	Professional Service	Fee	Payment	Adjustment	New Balance	Old Balance	Patient's Name	Distribution	
								Dr. Hayler	Dr. Meyer
TOTALS									

• Click **Finish** and continue to the next exercise.

Exercise 3

 Writing Activity—Preparing a Bank Deposit

15 minutes

Using the information you recorded in the day sheets in Exercise 2, you will now prepare a bank deposit (both front and back) for the accounts receivable for the day. Be sure the total on the deposit slip balances with the total of receivables on the day sheet.

1. Below, complete the front side of the deposit slip.

DEPOSIT SLIP

Clarion National Bank
90 Grape Vine Road
London, XY 55555-0001

Mountain View Clinic
4412 Broadway
London, XY 55555

Date: _____

_____
SIGN HERE IN TELLER'S PRESENCE FOR CASH RECEIVED

CASH			TOTAL
	Currency	$	
	Coin	$	
	Total Cash		$
CHECKS	See other side for detail		$
- CASH REC'D			$
NET DEPOSIT			$

2. Below, complete the back portion of the bank deposit slip. (*Note:* The bank number cannot be obtained from the day sheet. For the purposes of this exercise, use the check number as a substitute.)

BANK DEPOSIT DETAIL

PAYMENTS

BANK NUMBER	BY CHECK OR PMO		BY COIN OR CURRENCY		CREDIT CARD	
TOTALS						

CURRENCY		
COIN		
CHECKS		
CREDIT CARDS		
TOTAL RECEIPTS		
LESS CREDIT CARD $		
TOTAL DEPOSIT		
DEPOSIT DATE _____		

Exercise 4

Online Activity—Processing Credit Balances

 20 minutes

- From the Office Manager's area, click on the **Day Sheet** on the counter next to the computer keyboard. (*Note:* If you are at the office map, click on **Office Manager** and then click on the **Day Sheet**.)

1. Two patients listed on the day sheet have overpaid, resulting in a credit balance. What are the names of these two patients, and how much money should be refunded to each of them?

2. The day sheet indicates that _____ has already been sent a

   refund, but the refund for _____ still needs to be processed.

3. Using the blank check below, process the outstanding refund for payment.

173975			MOUNTAIN VIEW CLINIC 4412 Broadway London, XY 55555	173975 94-72/1224
DATE:			Date:	
TO:			Pay to the order of:	
FOR:				
BALANCE BROUGHT FORWARD			_____ Dollars	
DEPOSITS			Clarion National Bank *Member FDIC* 90 Grape Vine Road London, XY 55555-0001	
BALANCE				
AMT THIS CHECK				Authorized Signature
BALANCE CARRIED FORWARD				

‖⁕ 005503 ‖⁕ ⁙46782011 ‖⁕ 678800470

 • Click **Finish** to return to the manager's office.

Exercise 5

Online Activity—Maintaining Petty Cash Fund

30 minutes

- From the manager's office, click on the **Petty Cash Binder** (on the desk against the wall). (Note: If you are at the office map, click on **Office Manager** and select the **Petty Cash Binder**.)

1. Petty cash was used to pay for the mailing of a certified letter. What is the receipt number and date from this transaction?

2. On 5/1/07, the administrative medical assistant was asked to obtain soft drinks for an office celebration to be held that afternoon. She bought these at Sav-A-Grocery for the amount of $24.56. She also mailed a large package at the post office. The cost for mailing the package was $15.08. Using the form below, fill out the first petty cash voucher.

Date: _____ No.: _109_

Amount: [   ]

PETTY CASH VOUCHER

For: _____

Charge to: _____

_____

Approved by: Received by:

_____   _____

Authorized Signature

3. Now fill out the second petty cash voucher.

Date: _____   No.: __110__

Amount: [   ]

PETTY CASH VOUCHER

For: _____

Charge to: _____

_____

Approved by: Received by:

_____   _____

Authorized Signature

4. Using the completed petty cash vouchers from questions 2 and 3, update the petty cash log below. Be sure to distribute the expenses to the proper expense column.

NO.	DATE	DESCRIPTION	AMOUNT	OFFICE EXP.	AUTO.	MISC.	BALANCE
	2/16/2007	Fund Established (check #217)					200.00
101	2/24/2007	Certified Letter	3.74	3.74			196.26
102	3/1/2007	Staff Meeting/Lunch	24.60			24.60	171.66
103	3/6/2007	Coffee	4.32			4.32	167.34
104	3/8/2007	Tympanic Thermometer	38.00	38.00			129.34
105	3/8/2007	Parking Fee	6.00		6.00		123.34
106	4/1/2007	Staff Meeting/Lunch	27.43			27.43	95.91
107	4/13/2007	Miscellaneous Supplies	9.01	9.01			86.90
108	4/21/2007	Patient Birthday Cards	12.17	12.17			74.73

5. Office policy states that petty cash should be replenished when the amount falls below $50. Use the blank check below to replenish the petty cash fund to the full $200 balance as required by the office policy. Then, using the updated petty cash log in question 4, verify the petty cash fund balances by totaling all the columns and add this transaction to the log.

173976		
DATE:_____	MOUNTAIN VIEW CLINIC	173976
TO: _____	4412 Broadway	94-72/1224
FOR: _____	London, XY 55555	Date: _____
ACCOUNT No. _____	Pay to the order of: _____	
AMOUNT PAID $	_____ Dollars	

MOUNTAIN VIEW CLINIC
4412 Broadway
London, XY 55555

Date: _____

Pay to the order of: _____

_____ Dollars

Clarion National Bank
  Member FDIC
90 Grape Vine Road
London, XY 55555-0001

_____
Authorized Signature

||ꞏ 005503 ||ꞏ 446782011 ||ꞏ 678800470

➔ • Click **Finish** to return to the manager's office.

• Click the exit arrow and select **Return to Map**.

Exercise 6

Online Activity—Managing Accounts Payable

30 minutes

• Select any patient from the patient list; then click on **Reception** on the office map.

• Open the Incoming Mail window by clicking on the **Stackable Trays**. Review mail pieces 8 and 9.

1. Indicate whether each of the following statements is true or false.

   a. _____   When accounts payable arrive, the date for payment with discounts should be noted.

   b. _____   It really does not matter what day of the month an accounts payable payment is made, as long as it is paid before the next billing cycle.

   c. _____   Invoices should be marked with the date and check number, as well as the initials of the person preparing the check.

   d. _____   All accounts payables should be checked against invoices and packing slips before payment is made.

2. To correctly process and post the payment of the invoices (pieces 8 and 9 of the incoming mail), which of the following information does the accounts payable person need? Select all that apply.

_____ Invoice number

_____ Company name

_____ Name of customer service representative

_____ Date of check

_____ Account number

_____ Company address

_____ Company phone number

_____ Name of the company's bank

_____ Company bank account number

_____ Type of expense

_____ Amount of the check

_____ Invoice date

_____ Check number

- Click **Finish** to close the mail and return to the Reception desk.
- Click the exit arrow and select **Return to Map**.

Exercise 7

Online Activity—Reconciling a Bank Statement

30 minutes

In today's mail, the clinic's bank statement arrives. This can be found in the manager's office. She is extremely busy and asks that you take the time to reconcile the statement for her.

- On the office map, click on **Office Manager** to enter the manager's office. (*Note:* It is not necessary to select a patient to enter this area.)
- From the menu on the left, select **Bank Statement**.

1. a. Review the bank statement, comparing it against the check ledger below. On the ledger, check off each deposit, check, withdrawal, ATM transaction, or credit that is listed on the statement.
   b. If the statement shows any interest paid to the account or any service charges, bank fees, automatic payments, or ATM transactions withdrawn from the account that are not listed on the check ledger, make an entry for those items now and recalculate the account balance in the ledger.

No.	Date	Description	Payment/ Debit	Ref	Deposit/ Credit	Balance
1216	3/5/2007	Rocke Medical	$625.00			$9,264.35
1217	3/5/2007	Wal Store	$38.46			$9,225.89
1218	3/6/2007	Lorenz Equipment	$1,006.00			$8,219.89
1219	3/8/2007	Office Station	$199.43			$8,020.46
	3/10/2007	Dep. Daily Trans			$1,050.00	$10,833.46
1220	3/10/2007	West Electric	$93.99			$7,926.47
	3/12/2007	Dep. Daily Trans			$2,008.00	$9,934.47
1221	3/12/2007	Office Depot	$102.01			$9,832.46
1222	3/12/2007	Video Inc.	$49.00			$9,783.46
	3/15/2007	Dep. Daily Trans			$1,002.00	$11,835.46
1223	3/17/2007	Bonus	$200.00			$12,560.46
1224	3/17/2007	Bonus	$200.00			$12,360.46
1225	3/17/2007	Bonus	$200.00			$12,160.46
	3/20/2007	Dep. Daily Trans			$925.00	$12,760.46
1226	3/21/2007	Jamison Medical	$2,024.20			$10,136.26
1227	3/22/2007	Healthy Living Magazine	$32.95			$10,103.31
1228	3/22/2007	Greater London Electric	$422.00			$9,681.31
1229	3/24/2007	Office Station	$344.70			$9,336.61
1230	3/25/2007	Summer Oxygen	$230.99			$9,105.62
	3/27/2007	Dep. Daily Trans			$1,550.00	$10,655.62

2. Now complete the bank reconciliation worksheet below.

THIS WORKSHEET IS PROVIDED TO HELP YOU BALANCE YOUR ACCOUNT

1. Go through your register and mark each check, withdrawal, Express ATM transaction, payment, deposit or other credit listed on your statement. Be sure that your register shows any interest paid into your account, and any service charges, bank fees, automatic payments, or Express Transfers withdrawn from your account during this statement period.

2. Using the chart below, list any outstanding checks, Express ATM withdrawals, payments or any other withdrawals (including any from previous months) that are listed in your register but are not shown on this statement.

3. Balance your account by filling in the spaces below.

ITEMS OUTSTANDING		
NUMBER	**AMOUNT**	
TOTAL		

ENTER

The NEW BALANCE shown on this statement -------------------------------- $ _____ __

ADD

Any deposits listed in your register or $ _____ __
transfers into your account which are $ _____ __
not shown on this statement $ _____ __
                                           +$ _____ __

TOTAL---+ $ _____ __

CALCULATE THE SUBTOTAL --- $ _____ __

SUBTRACT

The total outstanding checks and
Withdrawals from the chart at the left --- $ _____ __

CALCULATE THE ENDING BALANCE

This amount should be the same as
The current balance shown in your
Check register -- $ _____ __

Procedural Coding (E&M and HCPCS)

Reading Assignment: Chapter 45—Medical Coding

Patients: Jean Deere, Wilson Metcalf, Teresa Hernandez

Learning Objectives:

- Explain the difference in levels of procedure codes.
- Indicate which codes are included in each section of the Current Procedural Terminology (CPT) manual.
- Assign correct CPT codes to services and/or procedures provided to selected patients.
- Identify when HCPCS level II codes should be used.
- Demonstrate how to locate an accurate HCPCS level II code.

Overview:

In this lesson you will learn the different levels of procedure codes as well as learn how to locate codes in the CPT Manual. You will have an opportunity to practice looking up diagnostic and procedure codes based on the patient documentation.

Exercise 1

Writing Activity—Coding Basics

5 minutes

1. Describe the difference in level I and level II Healthcare Common Procedure Coding System (HCPCS) codes.

2. Match the numeric codes below with the section of the CPT manual where they would be located.

	Section of the CPT Manual	**Numeric Codes**
_____	Anesthesia	a. 99201 to 99499
_____	Evaluation and Management	b. 90281 to 99199, 99500 to 99607
_____	Medicine	c. 80047 to 89356
_____	Pathology and Laboratory	d. 10021 to 69990
_____	Radiology	e. 70010 to 79999
_____	Surgery	f. 00100 to 01999, 99100 to 09140

3. When coding a medical history, how many levels are there to choose from?
   a. 1
   b. 2
   c. 3
   d. 4

4. List the types of medical history codes.

Exercise 2

Online Activity—Patient Medical Information for Correct Coding: Jean Deere

15 minutes

- Sign in to Mountain View Clinic.
- Select **Jean Deere** from the patient list.

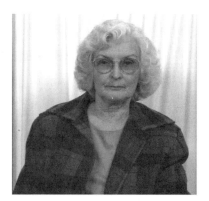

- Click on **Billing and Coding** on the office map.

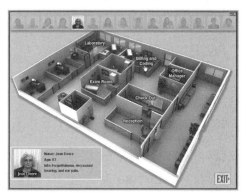

- Once you are in the Billing and Coding office, click on the **Encounter Form** (folder) on the desk to view the Encounter Form.

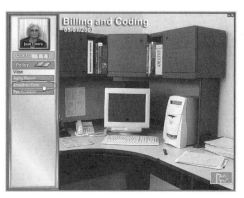

1. According to the Encounter Form, what procedures did Ms. Deere have today?

2. Ms. Deere is an established patient, and her office visit is considered a level IV visit. What number do the Evaluation and Management codes begin with?

3. The procedures provided to Ms. Deere today were (1) ear lavage, (2) UA dipstick, and (3) pulse oximetry. Below, match each procedure with the corresponding section of the CPT manual from which it should be coded.

Section of the CPT Manual	Procedure
_____ Medicine	a. Ear lavage
_____ Surgery	b. UA dipstick
_____ Pathology and Laboratory	c. Pulse oximetry

- Click **Finish** to close the Encounter Form.
- Click on the exit arrow and select **Return to Map**.
- On the office map, select **Exam Room**.
- Click on the **Exam Notes** folder on the left side of the counter to view Ms. Deere's Exam Notes.

4. Indicate whether the following statement is true or false.

_____ The procedures/services listed on the Encounter Form for Ms. Deere on this date match those documented in the Exam Notes.

- Click **Finish** to close Ms. Deere's chart.
- Click the exit arrow and select **Return to Map**.

Exercise 3

Online Activity—Patient Medical Information for Correct Coding: Wilson Metcalf

 15 minutes

- From the patient list, choose **Wilson Metcalf**. (*Note:* If you have exited the program, sign in again to Mountain View Clinic and select Wilson Metcalf from the patient list.)

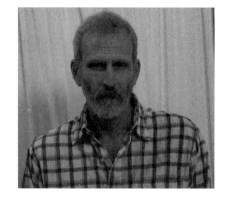

• Click on **Billing and Coding** on the office map.

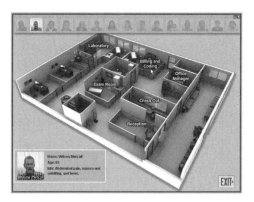

• In the Billing and Coding office, click on **Charts**.
• Click on the **Patient Medical Information** tab and choose **1-Progress Notes**.
• Review the Progress Notes before answering the following questions.

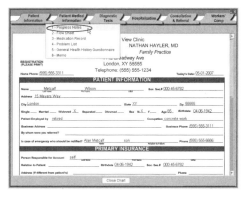

1. Were any laboratory tests completed for Mr. Metcalf on 5/1/07? If so, list each test.

2. Besides the examination, were any procedures performed on 5/1/07? If so, list and code each.

3. The use of modifiers in CPT coding can indicate that a service or procedure has been altered by some specific circumstance, but without changing its definition or code. Assume that Mr. Metcalf had a liver biopsy procedure that took more time than is typically required. Identify which modifier would be used in this example.

4. On the last day of his hospitalization, Mr. Metcalf underwent a needle biopsy of the prostate. What would be the correct CPT code for this procedure?
   a. 55700
   b. 55705
   c. 55720
   d. 55725

5. Indicate whether the following statement is true or false.

_____ Wilson Metcalf was discharged from the hospital on day 4. The physician spent a total of 45 minutes documenting the medical record and then discussing test results, prognoses, and medication requirements with the patient and his son. The correct CPT code for hospital discharge would be 99238.

→ • Close Mr. Metcalf's chart and **Return to Map**.

Exercise 4

Online Activity—CPT Coding Assignment

20 minutes

• From the patient list, choose **Teresa Hernandez**. (*Note:* If you have exited the program, sign back in and select Teresa Hernandez from the patient list.)

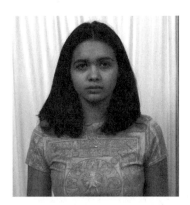

• Click on the **Billing and Coding** office.

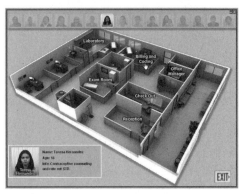

• Choose **Charts**, click on the **Patient Medical Information** tab, and select **1-Progress Notes**.

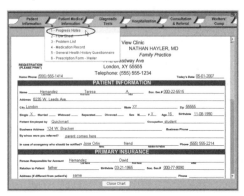

- Review the Progress Notes for 5/1/07.
- Click **Close Chart** and then click the **Encounter Form** on the desk.

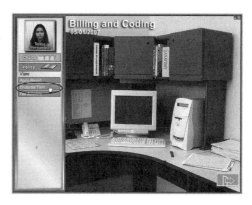

1. List and code all procedures/services that were performed for Teresa Hernandez on this date. (*Hint:* The urinalysis dipstick was performed by the manual method.)

2. Using your CPT manual, research the list of modifiers in Appendix A. Let's assume that Teresa is a level V established patient. Because of her multiple concurrent problems, her visit (including the examination, assessment, and counseling with the patient and her parents) took longer than usual—90 minutes. Is a modifier applicable to this situation? If so, what modifier should be used?

3. Teresa will return in 3 weeks for a Pap test. What CPT code should be used for this test? (*Hint:* The Bethesda method will not be used for this test.)

4. Indicate whether the following statement is true or false.

   _____ Teresa was given a prescription for a "seasonal oral contraceptive pack." This does not require a CPT code.

Diagnostic Coding

👓 **Reading Assignment:** Chapter 45—Medical Coding
  - Diagnostic Coding
  Chapter 46—Medical Insurance
  - Completing the Insurance Claim Form

Patients: Jose Imero, Kevin McKinzie

Learning Objectives:

- Describe the format and use of International Classification of Diseases, Ninth Revision, Clinical Modification (ICD-9-CM) codes.
- Demonstrate how fourth and fifth digits are used with ICD-9-CM codes.
- Demonstrate how to locate an accurate ICD-9-CM code.
- Demonstrate an understanding of the ICD-9-CM coding process by accurately coding patients' diagnoses to the greatest degree of specificity.

Overview:

In this lesson you will assign codes to various diagnoses using the latest edition of the ICD-9-CM codebook. You'll gain practice looking at the alphabetic and tabular sections of the codebook to verify the most appropriate code. You will also read patients' medical records and decide which codes to use for their diagnoses.

Please note that although Virtual Medical Office uses ICD-9 coding, many of these same exercises, perhaps with slight modifications, can be used to practice ICD-10 coding. Discuss expectations with your instructor.

Exercise 1

Writing Activity—Applying Accurate Codes to the Diagnoses Listed on the Encounter Form

75 minutes

1. Using the most recent edition of the ICD-9-CM codebook and the coding steps presented in the textbook, identify the correct diagnosis codes for each condition, diagnosis, or type of visit listed below.

Abscess _____

Acne _____

Alcohol abuse _____

Allergic reaction _____

Amenorrhea _____

Anemia _____

Anxiety _____

Annual GYN exam _____

Annual PE _____

Arrhythmia _____

Arthritis _____

Backache _____

Breast mass _____

Bronchitis _____

Bursitis _____

Chest pain _____

CHF _____

Conjunctivitis _____

COPD _____

Contraception _____

Cough _____

Depression _____

Dermatitis _____

Diarrhea _____

Dysmenorrhea _____

Ear impaction _____

Fatigue _____

Fever _____

Gastritis _____

Gastroenteritis _____

Gout _____

Headache _____

Hemorrhoids _____

Hypothyroidism _____

IBS _____

Low back pain _____

Lymphadenopathy _____

Nausea/vomiting _____

Otitis media _____

Pharyngitis _____

Pneumonia _____

Rectal bleed _____

Sinusitis _____

STD _____

Tendonitis _____

UTI _____

URI _____

Vaginitis _____

Well-baby/well-child _____

Weight loss _____

Exercise 2

Online Activity—Diagnostic Coding for Jose Imero

15 minutes

- Sign in to Mountain View Clinic.
- Select **Jose Imero** from the patient list.

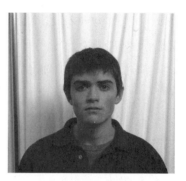

- Enter the **Exam Room** from the office map.

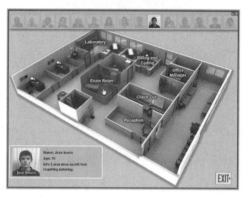

- In the Exam Room, select **Exam Notes** (under View).

1. Based on the Exam Notes, what is (are) the diagnosis(es) for this patient?

2. The first step in coding this diagnosis is to identify the _____ and

   locate it in the _____.

3. The main term of this patient's diagnosis is:
   a. laceration.
   b. left foot.
   c. plantar surface.
   d. inner aspect.

4. When you located the main term in the ICD-9-CM, what else were you instructed to do?

5. After completing the step you identified in question 4, what code(s) did you locate?

6. After cross-referencing the code(s) to the tabular section and coding the diagnosis to the greatest degree of specificity, what is the correct primary code that should be reported in Block 21 of the CMS-1500 claim form?

7. What is the rule for using E codes on an insurance claim?

8. When using a fifth digit in coding, where should the fifth digit be placed?

➤ • Close the **Exam Notes**.
   • Click on the exit arrow and select **Return to Map**.

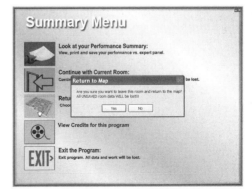

Exercise 3

Online Activity—Diagnostic Coding for Kevin McKinzie

 20 minutes

- Choose **Kevin McKinzie** from the patient list. (*Note:* If you have exited the program, sign back in to Mountain View Clinic and choose Kevin McKinzie from the patient list.)

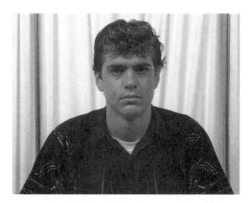

- On the office map, highlight and click on **Exam Room**.

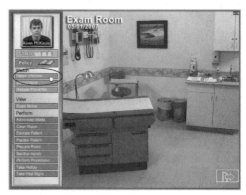

- In the Exam Room, select **Patient Interview** (under View).

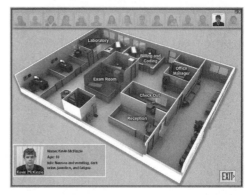

- At the end of the video, click **Close** to return to the Exam Room.
- Now select and review this patient's **Exam Notes**.

1. During the patient interview, what symptoms does the patient claim to have?

2. In the Exam Notes for this patient, what health problems does the physician document under "Impression"?

3. One entry in the Exam Notes under "Impression" is worded as "R/O hepatitis, mono." What is the rule about coding an entry like this?

4. When should an ICD-9-CM code be assigned to impressions documented as symptoms or worded as "rule out"?

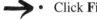 • Click **Finish** to close the Exam Notes. Click on the exit arrow and select **Return to Map**.
• Continuing with patient Kevin McKinzie, click on **Billing and Coding** on the office map.
• Click on **Encounter Form** and examine the diagnoses indicated for this patient.

5. Indicate whether each of the following statements is true or false.

   a. _____ The diagnoses indicated on Kevin McKinzie's Encounter Form are the same as those documented under "Impression" in the Exam Notes.

   b. _____ In Block 21 of the CMS-1500 form, the biller/coder should report the conditions/diagnoses documented in the patient's medical chart (Exam Notes) as opposed to those noted on the Encounter Form.

6. When the diagnoses listed on the Encounter Form are different from those documented in the medical record, the biller/coder should:
   a. report only the diagnosis codes noted on the Encounter Form.
   b. report only the diagnosis codes documented in the medical record.
   c. report both the diagnosis codes documented in the medical record and on the Encounter Form.
   d. report the discrepancy to the physician and ask for clarification regarding what specific diagnoses to code and report.
   e. insert an "addendum" to the medical record, adding the missing diagnosis codes from the Encounter Form.

7. Match each symptom or diagnosis with its correct ICD-9-CM code.

Symptom or Diagnosis	ICD-9-CM Code
_____ Dark urine	a. 780.79
_____ Nausea/vomiting	b. 787.01
_____ Fatigue	c. 788.9
_____ Asthma	d. 493.90
_____ Jaundice	e. 783.21
_____ Weight loss	f. 782.4

8. Note that "stomach pain" is not included in the Symptom or Diagnosis column in question 7. Why not?

9. Note that the physician *did* document "GI symptoms" under "Impression" in the Exam Notes. Can this condition be coded? Why or why not?

35

Medical Insurance

Reading Assignment: Chapter 46—Medical Insurance

Patients: Shaunti Begay, Louise Parlet, John R. Simmons, Janet Jones

Learning Objectives:

- Apply managed care policies and procedures to office billing and coding.
- Use third-party guidelines for preparing insurance claims and collecting copayments.
- Perform procedural coding.
- Perform diagnostic coding.
- Understand the importance of preparing a clean insurance claim form.

Overview:

In this lesson you will verify insurance for a new patient and consider how to resolve problems when a patient is not covered by her family's insurance plan for services rendered. You will learn about the requirements of patients being seen as part of a workers' compensation claim. You will assist a patient whose insurance requires a referral. Also discussed is the importance of accurately completing all insurance claim forms.

Exercise 1

Online Activity—Verifying Insurance for a New Patient

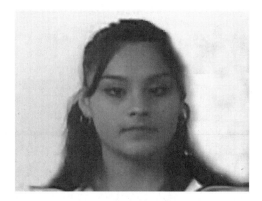

30 minutes

- Sign in to Mountain View Clinic.
- From the patient list, select **Shaunti Begay**.

- On the office map, highlight and click on **Reception**.

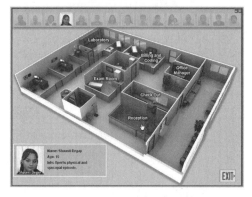

- At the Reception desk, click on **Policy** to open the office Policy Manual.

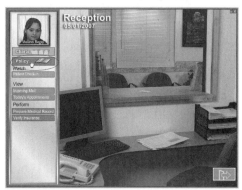

- Select the **Policy Manual**, type "17" in the search bar, and click the magnifying glass. This will take you to page 17 of the Policy Manual. Scroll up to adjust the page and read the policies that apply when patients have insurance coverage that is not accepted by the medical practice.

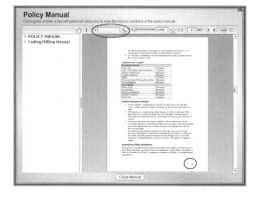

1. According to the Policy Manual, what process should be followed when a new patient schedules an appointment?

2. Why is it important for the medical assistant to verify *at the time the appointment is made* whether the office is a preferred provider with the patient's insurance?

→ • Scroll up to page 14 of the Policy Manual and read the section on Telephone Policies.

3. What does the Policy Manual state about collecting payments, copays, and percentages of charges for patient visits?

→ • Click **Close Manual** to return to the Reception desk.
  • Click on **Patient Check-In** to view the video of Shaunti's arrival at the clinic.

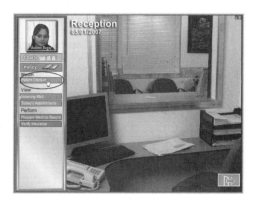

  • At the end of the video, click **Close** to return to the Reception desk.

→ • At the Reception desk, click on the **Insurance Card** on the window counter to obtain the required information for Shaunti's visit (clicking on the card opens the Verify Insurance window).

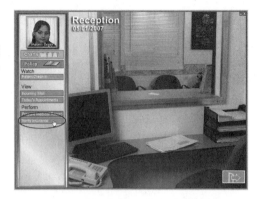

• Select the appropriate question to ask Shaunti's parents regarding her insurance; then review the Insurance Cards on the next screen.

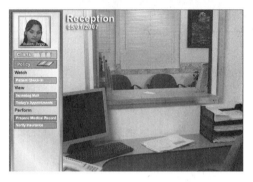

• Click **Finish** to return to the Reception desk.
• Click again on **Policy** to reopen the Policy Manual.
• From the menu on the left side of the screen, click on the arrow next to **Coding/Billing Manual** to view the additional headings for that section of the Policy Manual.
• Click the arrow next to **Financial Policy** and select **Accepted Insurance Carriers** from the list.

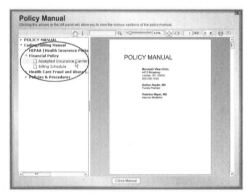

• Click **Close Manual** to return to the Reception desk.

4. Was Kristin correct in stating that Mountain View Clinic was not a participating provider for Shaunti's insurance plan?

5. What did Shaunti's mother say about the information she gave the receptionist regarding their insurance coverage when she made the appointment?

6. In hindsight, what steps, if taken by the medical assistant when the appointment was first made, would have prevented the confusion that occurred when Shaunti checked in today?

 • Click the exit arrow and select **Return to Map**.

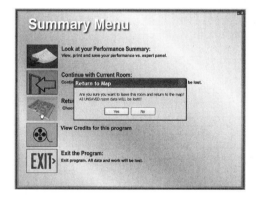

Exercise 2

 Online Activity—Obtaining a Referral for an Established Patient

 30 minutes

• Select **Louise Parlet** from the patient list. (*Note:* If you have exited the program, sign in again to Mountain View Clinic and select Louise Parlet from the patient list.)

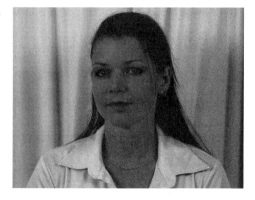

→ • On the office map, highlight and click on **Check Out**.

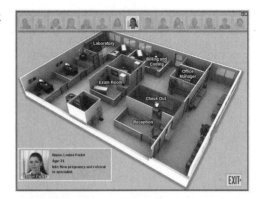

• At the desk, click on **Patient Check-Out** to view the video.

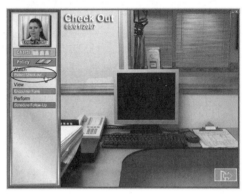

• At the end of the video, click **Close** to return to the desk.

1. Why is it important that the medical assistant help Ms. Parlet obtain approval from her insurance company for the referral to Dr. Lockett?

2. After receiving the precertification verification number, how should the medical assistant handle the verification number?

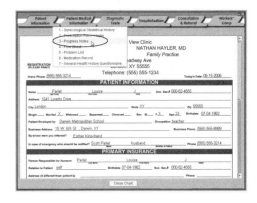

- Next, click on **Charts** to open Ms. Parlet's medical record.
- Under the **Patient Medical Information** tab, select **3-Progress Notes** and read Dr. Hayler's notes regarding the examination.

3. What instructions does Dr. Hayler give about the results of the lab work? How do these instructions affect the insurance coverage?

- Click **Close Chart** to return to the Check Out desk.
- Click the exit arrow and select **Return to Map**.

Exercise 3

Online Activity—Coding an Office Visit of a New Adult Patient

30 minutes

- Select **John R. Simmons** from the patient list. (*Note:* If you have exited the program, sign in again to Mountain View Clinic and select John R. Simmons from the patient list.)

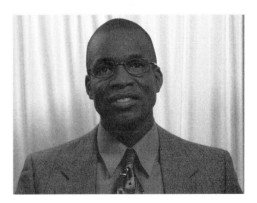

- On the office map, highlight and click on **Billing and Coding**.

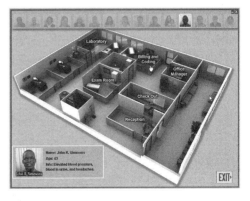

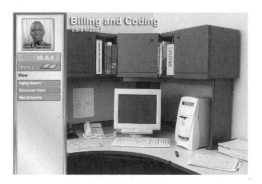

• At the Billing and Coding desk, click on the **Encounter Form** folder on the desk to view the diagnostic and procedural information for Dr. Simmons' visit.

1. In the ICD-9-CM section of the Encounter Form, which diagnoses are checked off for Dr. Simmons' visit?

2. Which of these diagnoses should receive an ICD-9-CM code? If there are any diagnoses that should not be coded, explain why not.

3. When should the home-obtained Hemoccult testing be billed and coded? Explain your answer.

• Click **Finish** to close the Encounter Form and return to the Billing and Coding desk.
• Click on **Charts** to open Dr. Simmons' medical record and select **5-Insurance Cards** from under the **Patient Information** tab.

4. Using the information on the insurance cards found in the medical record, what is the copay on the patient's insurance? What is the payment rate on the secondary insurance?

5. What is meant by PCP?

6. What is meant by POS?

- Click **Close Chart** to return to the Billing and Coding desk.
- Click the exit arrow and select **Return to Map**.

Exercise 4

Online Activity—Insurance Versus Workers' Compensation Claims

 15 minutes

- From the patient list, select **Janet Jones**. (*Note:* If you have exited the program, sign in again to Mountain View Clinic and select Janet Jones from the patient list.)

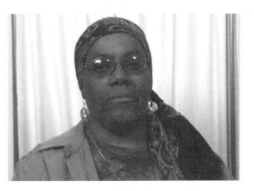

- On the office map, highlight and click on **Billing and Coding**.

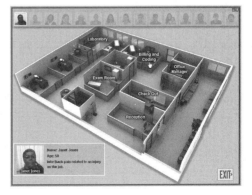

- Click on **Charts** to open Janet Jones' medical record.
- Next, click on the **Patient Information** tab.

1. You will notice that in Ms. Jones' medical record, there is no information about private insurance coverage. Why is this important for this case?

2. What information is needed for a workers' compensation claim that is *not* needed for a private insurance claim?

→ • Now click on the tab labeled **Workers' Comp**.

3. What information do you find under this tab in Ms. Jones' medical record?

4. If the workers' compensation carrier declares Ms. Jones' claim to be nonindustrial and refuses to pay it, is Mountain View Clinic required to write off the balance? (*Note:* Use your critical thinking skills to answer this question.)

Medical Office Management

👓 **Reading Assignment:** Chapter 48 — The Medical Assistant as Office Manager

Patient: Jose Imero

Learning Objectives:

- Describe the steps necessary for replenishing supplies.
- Discuss how having too many or too few supplies can affect the efficiency of the office.
- Decide which items to reorder and the amount to reorder.
- Explain the necessity of checking equipment for maintenance on a regular basis.
- Discuss the role of the medical assistant in suggesting new medical office equipment to the office manager.
- Identify unethical behaviors and apply critical thinking skills in suggesting ways to deal with a coworker's unprofessional actions.

Overview:

Ensuring the availability of supplies and equipment when needed is essential to the efficiency of the medical office practice. The proper inventory of supplies and equipment helps to ensure their ready availability. In some cases, it is more efficient to order supplies in larger quantities. The medical assistant who is also an office manager has the responsibility of making sure that the equipment ordered is the most currently used in the field. The first part of this lesson will focus on supplies and equipment and their importance to office efficiency.

The office manager also has the responsibility of ensuring that the medical office's employees are kind and courteous to patients and that they follow all office policies. The second part of this lesson will focus on questionable behaviors displayed by a Mountain View Clinic employee (observed in an earlier lesson). You will consider this employee's behavior and apply your critical thinking skills to decide what counseling is appropriate.

389

Exercise 1

Online Activity—Deciding When to Replenish Supplies

30 minutes

- Sign in to Mountain View Clinic.
- On the office map, highlight and click on **Office Manager** to enter the manager's office. (*Note:* You do not need to select a patient for this exercise.)

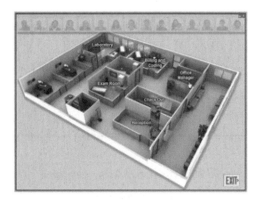

- Click on **Supply Inventory** to view the inventory records.

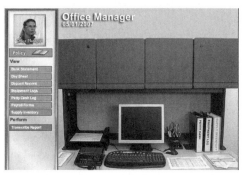

- To view the record for each item in the inventory, click on the corresponding tab headings.

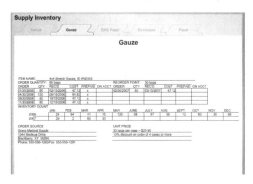

1. What is the reorder point for sutures?

2. Looking at the record from 2006, how many packages of sutures were previously used in May?

→ • Click on the tab heading for **Gauze** to view the inventory record.

3. What is the reorder point for gauze?

4. Looking at the record from 2006, how many bags of gauze were previously used in May?

5. The inventory for gauze is recorded in number of bags, but gauze can also be ordered by the case. How many bags are in a case?

6. What is the unit price? Does this represent the price per bag or the price per case?

7. What is the discount offered for ordering four or more cases of gauze?

8. Based on your review of the inventory supply sheet for gauze, should gauze be reordered? If so, why and how much? If not, why not? If you reorder, what will be the net amount of the purchase?

→ • Click on the tab heading for **EKG Paper** to view that inventory record.

9. When was the last order placed for EKG paper? How much was ordered?

10. When was this order received?

11. What is the reorder point for EKG paper?

12. How many packs of EKG paper are currently in inventory?

13. Should EKG paper be reordered now? If so, why? If not, why not? If you reorder, what quantity should be reordered?

14. The order for EKG paper is prepaid. What are some possible reasons for setting up a pre-paid order for this item? (*Note:* Use your critical thinking skills in answering this question.)

→ • Click on the tab heading for **Envelopes** to view that inventory record.

15. How often does the office normally order envelopes?

16. On February 28, 2007, the office ordered four more boxes of envelopes. When did this order arrive?

17. Why is there so much time between when the order is placed and when the order is received?

18. From what you see on the inventory form, do the envelopes need to be reordered? How could the office lower the price of the envelopes? Do you see a problem with the reorder point, and does this need to be changed? If the envelopes are reordered in bulk, what would be the price?

➜ • Click on the tab heading for **Paper** to view the inventory record for copier paper.

19. After examining the inventory supply card for copier paper, what is the cost for three cases?

20. What is the cost for ordering five cases?

21. How should the ordered supplies be handled when they arrive at the office?

➡ • Click **Finish** to return to the Office Manager area.

Exercise 2

Writing Activity—Maintaining and Suggesting Equipment

15 minutes

1. When filling the copier with paper, Cathy notices that the time for regular maintenance of the machine has passed, but the copier supplier representative has not been to the office. What should be Cathy's next step?

2. The toner cartridges are low, and Cathy sees a need for replenishing these. What should she do?

3. Armeeta has observed that not all patients with diabetes are using the same glucose meters at home. The physicians are asking that quality control be checked with patients more often. However, if the office does not have the same glucometers and supplies that some of the patients use at home, it is difficult to provide accurate patient teaching. What steps should Armeeta take to ensure that patient teaching is accurate and helpful to each patient?

4. Leah, as an administrative assistant, has found that the phone line for the medical office's fax machine is often busy when a fax needs to be received. Often the person attempting to send the fax calls to complain that it is difficult to get important information to the physicians. What steps should Leah take to demonstrate the need for another fax line for the medical office?

Exercise 3

 Writing Activity—Management Responsibilities and Staff

 20 minutes

- From the Office Manager area, click **Policy** to open the Policy Manual. (*Note:* If you have exited the program, sign in again, and click on Office Manager on the office map.)
- Select the **Policy Manual**, type "work ethics" in the search bar, and click the magnifying glass. Read this section, as well as the section on Professional Behavior.
- Click the exit arrow and select **Return to Map**.
- Select **Jose Imero** from the patient list and click on **Check Out**.
- At the Check Out desk, select **Patient Check-Out** (under Watch) and view the video.
- Pay close attention to the end of the video, when the medical assistants are interacting.

1. What are the ethical implications of Kristin asking another medical assistant for money from petty cash? What are your thoughts regarding Kristin asking Leah if the office manager really had to know?

 • Click **Close** to return to the Check Out desk.
- Click the exit arrow and select **Return to Map**.
- You may remember Kristin from earlier lessons. In one exercise, she was caring for Wilson Metcalf when he fainted in the waiting room. Let's look again at that video to refresh your memory.
- On the office map, select **Wilson Metcalf** from the patient list and click on **Reception**.
- Select **Patient Check-In** (under Watch) and view the video.
- Click **Close** to return to the reception desk.

2. What comment did Kristin make that was unprofessional?

3. Who was in the waiting room when Kristin made this comment?

4. Did Kristin violate office policy?

Critical Thinking Question

5. If you overheard a coworker make a statement such as the one Kristin made about Mr. Metcalf, what would you do?

Critical Thinking Question

6. If you were the office manager at Mountain View Clinic, how would you respond to this situations? Would you wait until Kristin's employment evaluation to discuss this with her, or would you address it immediately?

Critical Thinking Question

7. What should Kristin do to improve her behavior?